Establishing a Research-Friendly Environment

A HOSPITAL-BASED APPROACH

DOROTHY Y. BROCKOPP
PhD, MSN, RN, FAAN
Coordinator of Nursing and Allied Health Research Office, Baptist Health Lexington
Professor Emeritus, College of Nursing, University of Kentucky, Lexington

KAREN S. HILL
DNP, RN, NEA-BC, FACHE, FAAN
Chief Operating Officer/Chief Nursing Officer, Baptist Health Lexington
Editor-in Chief, *Journal of Nursing Administration*

ANDREW A. BUGAJSKI
PhD, BSN
Former Fellow/Research Consultant, Baptist Health Lexington
Current Assistant Professor, University of South Florida College of Nursing, Tampa

ALEXANDER J. LENGERICH
MS, EdS
Former Fellow/Research Consultant, Baptist Health Lexington
Current Doctoral Candidate, University of Kentucky Department of Educational,
School, & Counseling Psychology, Lexington

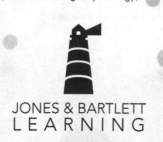

JONES & BARTLETT
LEARNING

World Headquarters
Jones & Bartlett Learning
5 Wall Street
Burlington, MA 01803
978-443-5000
info@jblearning.com
www.jblearning.com

Jones & Bartlett Learning books and products are available through most bookstores and online booksellers. To contact Jones & Bartlett Learning directly, call 800-832-0034, fax 978-443-8000, or visit our website, www.jblearning.com.

Substantial discounts on bulk quantities of Jones & Bartlett Learning publications are available to corporations, professional associations, and other qualified organizations. For details and specific discount information, contact the special sales department at Jones & Bartlett Learning via the above contact information or send an email to specialsales@jblearning.com.

Production Credits

VP, Product Management: David D. Cella
Director of Product Management: Amanda Martin
Product Manager: Teresa Reilly
Product Assistant: Christina Freitas
Production Manager: Carolyn Rogers Pershouse
Production Editor: John Fuller
Marketing Communications Manager: Katie Hennessy
Product Fulfillment Manager: Wendy Kilborn
Composition: S4Carlisle Publishing Services
Cover and Text Design: Kristin E. Parker
Director of Rights and Media: Joanna Gallant
Media Development Editor: Troy Liston
Rights & Media Specialist: John Rusk
Cover image: © gremlin/iStock/Getty Images
Printing and Binding: McNaughton & Gunn
Cover Printing: McNaughton & Gunn

Library of Congress Cataloging-in-Publication Data
Names: Brockopp, Dorothy Young, author. | Hill, Karen S., author. | Bugajski, Andrew A., author. | Lengerich, Alexander J., author.
Title: Establishing a research-friendly environment : a hospital-based approach / Dorothy Brockopp, Karen S. Hill, Andrew A. Bugajski, Alexander J. Lengerich.
Description: First edition. | Burlington, Massachusetts : Jones & Bartlett Learning, [2019] | Includes bibliographical references.
Identifiers: LCCN 2018034362 | ISBN 9781284141573 (paperback)
Subjects: | MESH: Nursing Research--organization & administration | Nursing Research--methods | Hospitals | Health Facility Environment | Models, Theoretical
Classification: LCC RT81.5 | NLM WY 20.5 | DDC 610.73072--dc23
LC record available at https://lccn.loc.gov/2018034362

6048

Printed in the United States of America
22 21 20 19 18   10 9 8 7 6 5 4 3 2 1

Contents

Preface vi

Acknowledgments viii

Reviewers ix

Introduction x

Chapter 1 Creating a Research-Friendly Environment in an Acute Care Setting . . . 1

Introduction 1

Support for Evidence-Based Practice 2

    Evidence-Based Practice: Benefits and Barriers 2

    Support for Evidence-Based Practice: Summary 3

The Healthcare System, Magnet, and Nursing Practice 4

    The Healthcare System 4

    Magnet Designation 4

    Nursing Practice 5

    The Healthcare System, Magnet, and Nursing Practice: Summary . . . 6

Evidence-Based Practice: Defining and Achieving 6

    Evidence-Based Practice: Defined . . . 7

    Achieving Evidence-Based Practice 7

    Gathering Evidence: An Example 9

    Evidence-Based Practice: Defining and Achieving: Summary 9

Methods Used to Base Practice on Evidence 10

    Evidence-Based Practice Projects . . . 13

    Quality Improvement 15

    The Research Process 17

    Methods Used to Base Practice on Evidence: Summary 17

Chapter 1 Summary 18

References 20

Chapter 2 Developing a Research-Friendly Environment: Strategies and Resources 23

Introduction 23

Conceptual Frameworks 25

    An Example of a Conceptual Framework 25

    Conceptual Frameworks: Summary 26

The Influence of Leadership 26

    Generous Leadership 27

    Generous Leadership: Activities 30

    The Influence of Leadership: Summary 33

Resources to Support a Research-Friendly Environment 33

    Research Consultants 33

    The Role of the Institutional Review Board (IRB) 36

    Searching the Literature: The Role of Librarians 37

    Resources Supporting the Research-Friendly Environment: An Example 38

    Funding for Research 39

Chapter Summary 39

References 42

Chapter 3 The Research-Friendly Environment Model 43

Introduction. 43
Exploration 45
    Caregiver Has an Idea 45
    Review of Relevant Literature. 47
    Initial Research Question 48
    Exploration: Summary. 50
Formulation 50
    Identify Variables and Measures 51
    Formulate an Intervention
      if Applicable. 53
    Procedure for Data
      Collection/Input. 54
    Formulation: Summary 56
Application. 56
    Institutional Review Board
      Approval 57
    Application: Summary. 57
Analysis 58
    Content Analysis 58
    Statistical Analysis: Descriptive. 59
    Statistical Analysis: Inferential
      Statistics. 59
Dissemination 61
    Delineated in an Organizational
      Policy Publication. 62
Chapter Summary 69
References 70

Chapter 4 Research Methods in a Research-Friendly Environment: An Overview. 75

Introduction. 75
Quantitative Research 76
    Assumptions Underlying
      Quantitative Research 77
    Quantitative Research
      Designs 77
    Descriptive Research Designs:
      Summary. 85
    Measurement 85

Sample Size and Selection. 87
Quantitative Research: Summary . . . 88
Qualitative Research 89
    Assumptions Underlying
      Qualitative Research. 89
    Types of Qualitative Research. 90
    Qualitative Research: Summary. 92
Chapter Summary 92
References 93

Chapter 5 Measurement: A Model for Instrument Development. 95

Introduction. 95
Measurement: A Model for
    Instrument Development 97
    Need for Measurement. 98
    Literature Review. 99
    Select Instrument from the
      Literature. 101
    Modify an Existing Instrument. 101
    Develop an Instrument. 103
    Administer the Instrument 116
Chapter Summary 118
References 120

Chapter 6 Statistical Analysis: Answering Questions 123

Introduction. 123
Computer Software. 124
Explanation of Statistical Terms
    and Concepts. 124
    Variables 125
    Independent and Dependent
      Variables 126
    Levels of Measurement. 127
    Statistical Significance. 128
    Means, Medians, and Modes 128
Type I and Type II Errors. 129
    Confidence Intervals 130
    Power Analysis 130
    Statistical Terms and Concepts:
      Summary. 131

Inferential Statistics 131
   Parametric and Nonparametric
      Statistics. 132
Descriptive Statistics .142
   Frequency Distribution 142
Chapter Summary 146
References 146

Chapter 7 Disseminating
Findings 149

Introduction. 149
Disseminating Findings: The Research
   Consultant's Role 151
   Internal Reports 151
   Abstracts. 151
Transforming Practice into Publication:
   A Research-Friendly Institution's
   Guide. 153
   Step 1: Preparing Early
      for Publication. 154
   Step 2: Evaluating Rigor
      of Design. 156
   Step 3: Developing the
      Manuscript 157
   Step 4: Selecting a Journal. 158
   Step 5: Collaborative Writing 160
   Step 6: Journal Submission 161
   Step 7: Response to Request
      for Revisions. 162
   Transforming Practice into
      Publication: A Research-Friendly
      Environment's Guide:
      Summary. 163
Disseminating Findings: The
   Journal's Perspective 163
   Letter or Email Message Is Sent
      to the Editor. 165
   Editor Responds to an Inquiry 165
   Editor's Decision to Reject or
      Forward for Review 165
   Role of Peer Reviewers 166
   Response to Authors: Editors
      and Reviewers. 166
   Requests for Revisions. 166

Chapter Summary 167
References 168

Chapter 8 Research-Friendly
Environments:
The Future 169

Introduction. 169
Magnet Designation: Increasing
   Expectations. 169
Patient Care: Changing Expectations 170
Hospital Culture: A Vision for
   the Future 170
Attitudes Toward Research:
   A New Direction 171
Use of Resources: A Recommendation
   for the Future 171
Administration: A Different Kind 172
The Profession of Nursing:
   Future Directions 175
Developing a Research-Friendly
   Environment: Hospital-Based
   Strategies 175
   The Neuroscience Nursing
      Research Center Fellowship
      Model. 177
   The Nursing Fellowship Program . . .178
   Research Training Program for
      Point-of-Care Clinicians 179
   The Research Consultation Model. . .179
   Requirements for Participation 180
   Developing a Research-Friendly
      Environment: Hospital-Based
      Strategies: Summary. 180
Caregiver Education: Future
   Strategies and Recommendations. . . .182
   The Nurse Scholars Strategy 184
   The Nurse Research Internship 185
Chapter Summary 186
References 187

Index. 189

Preface

My goal in collaborating with my coauthors to write this book is to encourage hospital-based caregivers, particularly those at the bedside, and students who hope to work in a hospital setting, to embrace the notion of conducting research in order to base practice on evidence. My "love affair" with evidence started when I was a faculty member at McMaster University, Ontario, Canada. I was fortunate to be there when David Sackett, MD, was on faculty. Known as the father of evidence-based practice, he set a stage that changed my view of nursing and health care. At that place and time, the randomized controlled trial was considered the gold standard and in many ways the only method for gaining meaningful and accurate information. I disagreed with that stance, however, and I took from that experience the desire to resolve patient-care problems by using the research process.

Given that basing patient care on evidence is a growing expectation across the globe, hospital-based nurses and other healthcare professionals are increasingly required to actively engage in research activities. Both government agencies and Magnet (a major designation of excellence in nursing care) have increasingly emphasized the need for evidence-based practice. As a result, Karen Hill, Chief Operating Officer/Chief Nursing Officer at Baptist Health Lexington, asked me to join the organization on a half-time basis and develop a research program. In addition to my love for research, I learned during 30 years of teaching undergraduate and graduate nursing students that nurses at the bedside were capable of developing and conducting studies. Eight years as a half-time research consultant at a university hospital and 10 years at a community hospital in the same position have taught me that, in general, hospital-based clinicians make superb researchers. At Baptist Health Lexington, I wanted to establish a culture that would encourage and support all caregivers at the bedside, regardless of educational preparation, to design and conduct studies and also publish their findings.

Karen and I wanted more than a research program. We wanted the hospital environment to change. Our goal was to develop a research-friendly environment that would welcome ideas for projects from any caregiver, provide support for those ideas to be operationalized, and acknowledge all outcomes. As a result, over the past 8 years, caregivers at the hospital have published 51 articles in peer-reviewed journals. Thirty-one of the first authors are prepared at the graduate level, 10 at the baccalaureate level. Two associate degree–prepared nurses completed studies and published findings in peer-reviewed journals. Twenty-six caregivers prepared at the baccalaureate level are coauthors.

The strategy of identifying caregivers with advanced degrees as the only individuals who may conduct research is unlikely to meet the need for evidence to support changes in health care. In addition, it is the caregiver at the bedside who best understands patient care problems that need to be resolved. With that in mind, we have developed an environment that has displaced the notion that only individuals with graduate degrees can conduct research. The following pages explain and clarify the reasons why hospital-based caregivers need to be involved in research, how hospitals can develop a research-friendly environment, and what knowledge is necessary for research consultants and caregivers to actively move toward evidence-based practice. This text also emphasizes the important role leadership plays in supporting the generosity needed to attain these outcomes.

—Dorothy Brockopp

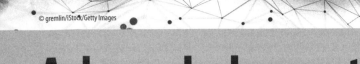

Acknowledgments

My coauthors and I would like to thank the hospital administrators at Baptist Health Lexington for making this research-friendly environment (RFE) become a reality. Their willingness to envision a different future for hospital employees in relation to their involvement in research and their courage to support considerable environmental change is responsible for the successes described in this text.

—*Dorothy Brockopp*

Reviewers

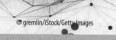

Kristin Ashford, PhD, WHNP-BC, FAAN
Associate Dean of Undergraduate
  Faculty and Interprofessional
  Education
University of Kentucky, College
  of Nursing
Lexington, KY

Evelyn Brewer, PhD(c), MSN, RN
Less-McRae College
Banner Elk, NC

Theresa G. Buxton, PhD, RN, CNE
Regis University
Denver, CO

Jill Dewlander, MSN, RN, APRN, ACCNS-AG,
CCRN-CSC
Clinical Nurse Specialist
Sentara RMH Medical Center
Timberville, VA

Heather Galang, MSN, RN-BC, CNL
Sentara Healthcare
Norfolk, VA

Kathleen Hall, PhD, APRN, GNP-BC
Assistant Professor of Nursing
Colorado Mesa University
Grand Junction, CO

Susan Mullen Kaplan, PhD, RN, CCRP
Sentara Norfolk General Hospital
Norfolk, VA

Kelley Kostich, MS, BSN, RN, NE-BC
Program Manager, Professional
  Practice and Development
Missouri Baptist Medical Center
St. Louis, MO

Sarah A. Mowry Lackey, DNP, APRN, CCNS
Cone Health
Winston-Salem, NC

Patricia McAllen, PhD, RN, CNE
Dean/Chief Operating Officer/
  Professor of Nursing
Mercy College of Ohio
Youngstown, OH

Sherri Mendelson, PhD, CNS, RNC, IBCLC
Providence Holy Cross Medical Center
Mission Hills, CA

Katherine Quartuccio, DNP, RN
Associate Professor
State University of New York at Delhi
Delhi, NY

David Sharp, PhD, MSc, MA
Professor of Nursing
Mississippi College
Clinton, MS

Cheryl Swanson, PhD, RN
Anna Vaughn College of Nursing
Oral Roberts University
Tulsa, OK

Cynthia Wachtel, MSN, RN
Nursing Faculty
Siena Heights University
Adrian, MI

Shu-Yi Wang, PhD, RN, CNS
Regis University
Denver, CO

Susan A. Winslow, DNP, RN, NEA-BC
Sentara Healthcare
Norfolk, VA

Kristen Zulkosky, PhD, RN, CNE
Pennsylvania College of Health
  Sciences
Lancaster, PA

Introduction

▶ Developing a Research-Friendly Environment: Engaging Caregivers

The emphasis in health care on evidence-based practice, practitioners' desire to provide optimal patient care, and criteria for Magnet designation (an international designation of nursing excellence) provided the motivation to write a text that would detail how caregivers can increasingly be involved in obtaining evidence for practice. The term *caregiver,* in this text, refers to those healthcare professionals who contribute to the provision of patient care in a hospital setting. A changing healthcare environment requires these individuals to continuously identify patient-care issues and attempt to design alternatives to present practices. Evidence suggests that caregivers want to provide the best care possible (Bugajski et al., 2017), and Magnet designation requires that nurses actively participate in activities such as research that will improve patient care (American Nurses Credentialing Center, 2013).

Initiating and maintaining hospital-based research programs that emphasize the involvement of caregivers at the bedside are the focuses of this text. A goal of the text is to provide information gained over a 10-year period at a 391-bed Magnet-designated community hospital that could assist others to initiate and maintain research activities within their institutions. Guidance is provided for caregivers and hospital administrators who want to encourage participation in research. In this research-friendly environment (RFE), the desired outcome of participating in research is to discover information that will lead to the provision of optimal patient care.

Strategies for developing RFEs as well as basic research methods are presented. Reasons for developing RFEs, necessary resources, and how to conduct research and disseminate findings are addressed. Using this text as a guide, an RFE can be initiated that will enable caregivers to identify patient-care issues and conduct studies in order to resolve those issues. Findings may be generalizable across institutions or applicable to their own setting.

For those studies that do not result in generalizable findings, information gained may motivate others to design studies on the same topic, that can be generalized to other settings. In this RFE, publication of results of caregiver-initiated research is assumed. Both qualitative and quantitative methods are used, although more quantitative than qualitative studies are conducted. In relation to quantitative research, descriptive and experimental designs are used. Experience has shown that both approaches can result in information that can lead to meaningful changes in practice.

For example, a descriptive study that was conducted using strategies described in this text has provided useful information for the institution. Findings were published, and the article has been frequently cited in the literature. This study provided information regarding factors that influence women to breastfeed and also tested an intervention that could encourage women to breastfeed (Kjelland et al., 2014). Although results could not be considered directly applicable to other hospital settings, caregivers at other institutions could conduct a randomized controlled trial with the possibility that results could be generalized to other hospitals. Meanwhile, based on findings, changes were made at this institution. The timeline for nurses to talk to new mothers regarding breastfeeding was modified, giving nurses more flexibility to have a discussion regarding breastfeeding at their convenience. Through publication, information was conveyed to other caregivers, including primary care and women's health providers who are concerned about the diminishing number of women who are breastfeeding their newborn infants.

The projected audience for this text includes individuals who are studying to become caregivers, plan to provide patient care in an acute care setting, or are presently employed at a hospital. Educators might also find this text useful. In order to prepare students to participate in hospital-based research, educational programs may need to change. Basic research skills beyond reviewing the literature would facilitate new graduates moving quickly into a role that includes research activities. Chapter 8 of this text, Future Directions, includes a proposed syllabus for an undergraduate course that would prepare nurses to participate in research.

There are many approaches to preparing caregivers to engage in hospital-based research activities. Designing a syllabus that would require students to participate in each component of the research process, working with researchers on a specific project in order to meet program requirements, and bringing researchers into the classroom to talk with students about their studies are three possibilities. Attitudes would also need to be addressed. Teaching undergraduate students that they can engage in research activities beyond reading the literature would prepare them to actively participate in and lead projects in their clinical settings.

In addition to caregivers, this text is written to assist hospital administrators to develop an RFE. Administrators interested in pursuing or maintaining Magnet designation could find the information provided in this text useful in developing an environment that supports and encourages research. Magnet designation requires nurses' participation in research activities. In order to encourage caregivers to participate in research, supportive, active leadership is essential. The task is to modify the culture so that caregivers are comfortable designing and conducting research projects.

Experienced caregivers in both nursing and allied health, as well as undergraduate students in clinical programs, can also benefit from the content in this text. Given the emphasis on providing evidence-based care from the government, professional organizations, and many hospital administrators, conducting research at the caregiver level is increasingly important. New graduates need skills that have not been a priority in the past. In addition to new skills related to research, attitudes need to change. Embracing the idea of conducting studies to obtain meaningful information to support patient care, rather than believing necessary knowledge and skills are out of reach, needs to be addressed in the hospital setting.

Caregivers with graduate degrees have traditionally been expected to participate in research activities. The information provided in this text can assist caregivers at all levels of educational preparation to participate in the development of an environment that supports and encourages research. Nurses in particular need to become involved in developing a hospital-based research program. In addition to

Magnet designation, nurses constitute the largest group of employees in a hospital setting and have continuous relationships with patients. Hospital administrators, particularly chief nursing officers, are key to involving nurses in research activities.

The text consists of eight chapters that present the following: reasons for developing a hospital-based research program emphasizing caregiver-initiated research, strategies and resources used at one hospital to develop a successful RFE, a model designed to guide caregivers to conduct research, and basic skills and knowledge necessary for caregivers to design and conduct studies and publish their findings. Basic skills and knowledge include reviewing the literature; designing a research question; developing interventions; designing studies; selecting, modifying, or developing instruments; applying to the institutional review board; collecting data; analyzing data; and disseminating findings. The chapter on dissemination of findings provides strategies to help caregivers publish the results of their studies. Adoption of practice changes suggested by results of studies conducted is guided by principal investigators working with administration. These strategies have resulted in an acceptance rate of 97% by peer-reviewed journals. In addition, future directions in relation to hospital environments, nursing and allied health education, and the profession of nursing are described in the last chapter. To support content, examples of studies conducted in this RFE are presented.

▸ References

American Nurses Credentialing Center. (2013). *2014 Magnet application manual.* Silver Springs, MD: Author.

Bugajski, A., Lengerich, A., Marchese, M., Hall, B., Yackzan, S., Davies, C., & Brockopp, D. (2017). The importance of factors related to nurse retention: Using the Baptist Health nurse retention questionnaire, Part 2. *Journal of Nursing Administration, 47*(6), 308–312. doi:10.1097/nna .0000000000000486

Kjelland, K., Corley, D., Slusher, I., Moe, K., & Brockopp, D. (2014). The Best for Baby Card: An evaluation of factors that influence women's decisions to breastfeed. *Newborn and Infant Nursing Reviews, 14*(1), 23–27. doi:10.1053/j.nainr.2013.12.007

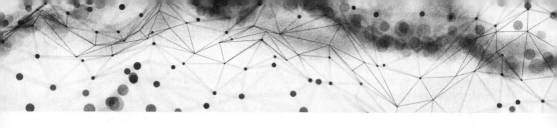

CHAPTER 1

Creating a Research-Friendly Environment in an Acute Care Setting

"Evidence-based practice provides a framework for a specific clinical way of life."

— **Porter-O'Grady**, 2010

▶ Introduction

The emphasis throughout health care on evidence-based practice (EBP) is a major reason underlying the development of caregiver-initiated research programs. In this chapter, the movement toward EBP in hospital settings is described. In addition, EBP is defined and factors influencing the direction health care is taking in regard to basing care on evidence are addressed. These factors include changes in the healthcare system, requirements for Magnet designation, and changing expectations of nurses that make active participation in research a challenge.

Examples of actions taken to support research, as well as studies conducted by healthcare professionals, are included in this chapter and throughout the text. All research activities described are a reflection of the research-friendly environment (RFE) that has been developed at Baptist Health Lexington (BHLex), a 391-bed community hospital located in the southeastern United States.

In addition, three methods for obtaining evidence to support evidence-based care are addressed: EBP projects, quality improvement projects, and studies based on the research process. While these approaches to obtaining evidence differ from one another, they also overlap and together can provide meaningful information.

For example, questions can arise as a result of EBP projects and quality improvement projects that can then be addressed using the research process.

▶ Support for Evidence-Based Practice

The major reason for developing an environment that supports research is the need and—at times—a requirement to base practice on evidence. Other reasons include the increasing acuity of inpatients, the realization that care based on evidence is both cost-effective and optimal, and hospitals' desire to be Magnet designated. As the patient acuity level in hospitals increases, new approaches to care are needed. Basing care consistently on evidence has been shown to diminish the cost of patient care and decrease morbidity (McClelland & Albert, p. 3,4, 2016). The philosophical underpinnings of Magnet designation support EBP, and that designation has become increasingly important to hospitals.

Evidence-Based Practice: Benefits and Barriers

In addition to improving patient care, hospital-based research conducted by caregivers can benefit an acute care institution in a number of ways. According to nurse leaders at the Cleveland Clinic (McClelland & Albert, 2016), hospital-based nursing research programs can be highly beneficial. They suggest that involving healthcare professionals in conducting research can improve clinical outcomes, offer opportunities for interdisciplinary work, and increase patient and staff satisfaction. An example of improved clinical outcomes occurred at BHLex related to falls. Inpatient falls decreased following the design and use of the Baptist Health High Risk Falls Assessment (Corley et al., 2014). Staff satisfaction related to conducting research was also apparent at this institutiton. Comments reported in BHLex's annual report (Baptist Health Lexington, 2014) by two nurses reflect their satisfaction with the support provided by the institution that enabled them to conduct research (see **BOX 1-1**).

 BOX 1-1 Nurse Champions

Melanie Thompson, RN, ADN

Melanie, a nurse in the hospital's preoperative area, wrote the following: "As an associate degree–prepared nurse, research was foreign to me. With support from the Medical Library, Nursing Research Office, and the IRB, I was able to successfully complete a research project to improve patient care in my department and later publish my findings in the *Journal of Radiology Nursing*. I would like to extend my appreciation to all these individuals, for helping me reach new heights as a clinical nurse at this wonderful facility!" (Baptist Health Lexington, 2014).

Holly Weyl, RN, BSN, OCN

Holly, a gastrointestinal nurse navigator, wrote, "It has been such an incredible honor and learning experience to conduct my first research study and publish my work in the *Clinical Journal of Oncology Nursing*. Our success was accomplished through a team effort with the support from the Medical Library, IRB, and Nursing Research Office. It means a lot to work at a hospital that supports nurses who are passionate about improving patient care" (Baptist Health Lexington, 2014).

The aging population and the introduction of complex treatments across diagnoses require nurses and other healthcare professionals working at the bedside to become more involved in obtaining and evaluating evidence. The associated increase in comorbidities from a rapidly aging population, higher patient acuity levels in the hospital setting, and increasing cost of hospital-based care require new and innovative practice strategies (McClelland & Albert, 2016; River, Cohen, & Counsell, 2006). Given these issues, obtaining evidence that can be consistently used to guide care can be beneficial to hospitals.

Despite the increased emphasis on developing new evidence-based approaches to care, involving clinicians at the bedside in strategies that will produce evidence remains a challenge. Healthcare professionals often report having little time and energy to design and conduct research projects due to a heavy workload and increasing responsibilities (Kelly, Turner, Speroni, McLaughlin, & Guzetta, 2013). Nurses, in particular, are expected to do more within the same time frame. Sicker patients often mean greater nursing responsibilities.

Regarding the skills necessary to actively participate in nursing research, it is common practice to include one three-credit course on research in undergraduate nursing curricula. In general, these courses are not designed to encourage or enable graduates to actively participate in designing and conducting studies; instead, students are taught to read and evaluate the literature and apply findings to their practice (Tingen, Burnett, Murchison, & Zhu, 2009). In addition, it is likely that literature shared with students is, for the most part, written by individuals with doctoral degrees.

While this approach to research at the undergraduate level is productive in many ways, more is expected from new graduate nurses at this point in time. Teaching basic research skills at the undergraduate level could assist nurses to add participation in studies to an already busy patient care schedule. Having to learn these skills in the hospital setting can become a burden for both caregivers and administrators who need to provide learning opportunities.

Support for Evidence-Based Practice: Summary

The majority of studies conducted in this RFE reflect interdisciplinary activity. In addition, anecdotal data suggest that increased staff satisfaction is a result of support for research activities. Of the 51 projects conducted in 2016, approximately one-third were led by teams of individuals from multiple disciplines. Authors of 31 of the 45 manuscripts published in peer-reviewed journals (2011–2017) represent multidisciplinary teams of investigators. Changes in practice based on project outcomes tend to occur prior to publication, and the number of citations of published articles suggests that changes may be occurring nationally.

Barriers that caregivers encounter in relation to conducting research, such as lack of time, limited resources, fear of engaging in the research process, and a dearth of research skills, are frequently present in hospital settings. Overcoming these barriers can lead to engagement across disciplines, job satisfaction and improved patient outcomes. Lack of time is frequently addressed in this RFE by unit managers who support research and assist investigators to work as a team and limit responsibilities for individuals. Resources can be provided at a modest cost, and attitudes toward engaging in research activities can be modified. Research skills can be taught to caregivers as they work on their projects.

▶ The Healthcare System, Magnet, and Nursing Practice

Changes in the healthcare system and a desire among hospitals for Magnet designation have motivated hospital administrators to encourage healthcare providers to participate in research activities that will lead to EBP. In addition, a need to diminish the cost of in-hospital care through efficient use of resources, increase provider work satisfaction, and provide optimal patient care are goals that drive the search for evidence. Unfortunately, increased responsibilities and expectations of nurses providing inpatient care can be barriers to including them in the search for evidence.

The Healthcare System

The use of evidence as a basis for practice has been influenced by changes in the healthcare system in the United States. Since the implementation of the Patient Protection and Affordable Care Act (ACA, 2010), efforts have been made to increase the efficiency of the healthcare system by making care more effective and less costly. Increased patient satisfaction, improved outcomes, and decreased cost have been identified as goals at all levels of health care (Berwick, Nolan, & Whittington, 2008). In order to meet these goals, the use of evidence as a component of clinical decision making has become increasingly important. For example, a report from the Institute of Medicine (IOM, 2011) stated that by 2020, 90% of clinical decisions should be based on accurate information from available evidence. This focus on EBP has motivated nurses and other healthcare providers to review relevant research and conduct projects aimed toward improving patient care. Although additional changes in the healthcare system may occur over time, because efficiency of care has been so closely linked with basing practice on evidence, the pursuit of evidence is likely to continue.

Magnet Designation

In addition to an emphasis on EBP, another important change for hospitals globally is the increasing interest in Magnet designation. In 1991, the American Nurses Credentialing Center (ANCC) introduced the Magnet Hospital Recognition Program for Excellence in Nursing Services. As of 2017, 442 hospitals have received Magnet designation in the United States, with 6 more internationally. In addition to reflecting the provision of outstanding patient care, Magnet designation is often viewed by hospital administrators as a means to attract strong practitioners from all fields and promote market excellence. Over time, elected officials and members of the public have also become aware of the importance of Magnet designation (Steinbinder & Scherer, 2016). As the public becomes aware of differences in levels of patient care at specific institutions, individuals will choose Magnet-designated hospitals when possible. It is clear that recognition of institutional excellence is a goal of many hospitals worldwide.

To receive this designation, institutions must be willing to examine past practices and attempt to discover new, innovative approaches to care (ANCC, 2008). Continuous improvement in the quality of care provided is inherent in the Magnet philosophy. When applying for Magnet designation, hospitals must provide in-depth data on all aspects of nursing performance and patient care, as well as evidence that nurses are active participants in research. In 2016, BHLex was designated for the third time and was cited as an exemplar in relation to nursing research. A 10-year journey that began with no caregiver-initiated studies and no publications resulted in approximately 40 ongoing projects a year and 30 publications.

Caregivers have learned that publication of their work is a desirable outcome. An example of the change in culture regarding research activities occurred when a bedside nurse was asked by a Magnet visitor what the final outcome would be for the poster on the wall describing a study conducted on that unit; she replied, "Publication, of course." The initial fear among nurses with undergraduate degrees of writing a manuscript has diminished over time. As their colleagues met with success, more nurses became interested in conducting research, including efforts to publish their findings.

As a result of Magnet's emphasis on providing optimal patient care based on evidence, this designation has played a major role in motivating nurses to conduct research. This emphasis on EBP has also motivated hospital administrators to provide resources to assist nurses to participate in research activities. The requirements for designation as a Magnet hospital include infrastructures that enable and support nurses to access evidence related to patient care, active involvement in conducting research, and documentation that clinical practice is based on evidence. Hospitals are challenged to create an environment that motivates nurses to understand the importance of basing practice on evidence, supports research activities, and acknowledges the contributions of nurses who are actively engaged in pursuing evidence (ANCC, 2013). As hospitals strive to achieve and maintain Magnet designation, they will be required to develop environments that support research activities, including dissemination of findings.

Nursing Practice

Nurses constitute the largest number of professional staff in acute care settings. They engage in continuous relationships with their patients and are an invaluable resource in terms of identifying unmet patient needs. Barriers to nurses' systematically examining patient needs or problems include caring for sicker patients with more complex problems, the expenditure of more time and energy caring for each patient, negative attitudes toward research, and lack of leadership that supports nurses when they question present practices and want to find answers. Another barrier is a simple lack of time; for example, as a result of fast-paced changes in technology, nurses are required to spend already limited time and energy on tasks other than patient care, such as in learning new approaches to documentation and communication (McClelland & Albert, 2016).

Although a desire for lifelong learning has traditionally been a prerequisite for entrance into nursing, the pace at which nurses must learn has dramatically increased (Benner, Sutphen, Leonard, & Day, 2010). Asking nurses to base their practice on evidence while also requiring more of nurses in terms of patient care mean that hospitals must develop an environment that supports and enables nurses to be involved in research activities. The RFE at BHLex was designed to develop a culture that would provide support for research activities, acknowledge success in the area of research, and encourage staff at all levels to base patient care on evidence.

In addition to the issues already discussed, there is a serious shortage of nurses. The rate of growth between 2014 and 2024 within the nursing profession is projected at 16% (Bureau of Labor Statistics, 2016). That rate of growth will not meet the need for nurses. In order to attract and retain nurses, it is necessary for hospital administrators to engage nurses at their level of expertise in all areas and provide as much support as possible. Although not essential to developing an environment that supports research, in this RFE, nurses and other healthcare professionals have support from librarians, research consultants, and institutional review board coordinators (see Chapter 2).

In the Research Friendly Environment Model (RFEM) described in Chapter 3, nurses and other clinicians at the bedside are viewed as exceptional resources for not only identifying patient-care problems but also for suggesting alternative interventions. Providing support for them to test their ideas can be a goal of administration and research consultants. Given that most clinicians at the bedside want to improve patient care, providing opportunities for them to resolve issues they identify as they care for patients can increase work satisfaction and retention, which in turn can make hospitals that espouse these values more attractive to nurses seeking employment.

Traditionally, nurses at the bedside have not been expected to actively participate in research activities. However, experienced nurses are an untapped resource in terms of identifying patient care problems. In general, expectations regarding their involvement in investigating patient-care issues have been limited to reading, evaluating, and applying findings of published studies. In general, undergraduate courses in research have supported this view. Tradition holds that graduate degrees, preferably a doctorate, are required for principal investigators and first authors of data-based articles (Hedges & Williams, 2014).

Given appropriate resources and administrative support, nurses and other clinicians at the bedside can be principal investigators on research projects aimed at providing optimal patient care based on evidence. In this environment, 29 nurses at the bedside have been first authors or coauthors on peer-reviewed, data-based publications (2008 to present) leading to practice changes. Each study conducted in this RFE has focused on an issue raised by an experienced practicing caregiver.

The Healthcare System, Magnet, and Nursing Practice: Summary

For reasons related to the cost of health care, patient morbidity and mortality, and patient and provider satisfaction, the search for evidence to support practice will continue. How nurses and other providers can engage in activities to reach the goal of basing care on evidence is unclear. To move forward in a way that enables clinicians at the bedside to be actively involved in research, changes may need to occur in both educational and hospital settings. Basic research skills may need to be taught to undergraduates, and hospitals may need to create a culture that encourages caregivers to initiate research projects. Confusion regarding what constitutes EBP should also be addressed. A clear definition of what constitutes EBP would assist caregivers to engage in a search for evidence. Differences between EBP and EBP projects are clarified in the next section.

▶ Evidence-Based Practice: Defining and Achieving

Developing an understanding of EBP as presented in the literature is an important first in developing hospital-based environments that encourage research. At present, there is some confusion as to whether EBP is an outcome or the result of a method—EBP projects—used to change practice based on evidence. As an outcome, EBP refers to care that is based on data that have been analyzed and from which conclusions have been derived. As a method, EBP is a set of steps that enables providers to improve practice based on clinical expertise and available research. For purposes of this text, EBP is viewed as an outcome, and those steps taken to change practice are seen as a predetermined method. The method is described as conducting EBP projects.

Evidence-Based Practice: Defined

EBP is often defined within nursing as a process that includes consideration of nursing theory as well as practitioners' clinical expertise in considering and evaluating the delivery of nursing care (Scott & McSherry, 2009). The medical literature defines evidence-based medicine as "the conscientious, explicit and judicious use of current best evidence in making decisions about the care of individual patients" (Sackett, 1996, p. 1). In both cases, practice based on evidence refers to a process that focuses on improving patient care in relation to efficiency and outcomes. It is a complex process that requires an ongoing interest in questioning present approaches to clinical decision making.

Achieving Evidence-Based Practice

Basing practice on evidence not only leads to improved care but can also diminish cost by requiring healthcare professionals to intervene on a more consistent basis. Leaders in both medicine (Sackett, Straus, Richardson, Rosenberg, & Haynes, 2000) and nursing (Mallach & Porter-O'Grady, 2010) have actively supported the use of EBP across professions. They describe EBP as a process of clinical decision making that uses the best available evidence, incorporates clinical expertise in providing care, and considers patient and family preferences as well as available resources (DiCenso, Guyatt, & Ciliska, 2005). EBP is associated with cost savings, diminished length of stay for patients, and decreased admissions to the hospital (Jones et al., 2015; Wyer et al., 2016). While most healthcare professionals would agree that providing optimal care for patients is their goal, there are concerns regarding the present emphasis on EBP.

One of the concerns is the belief that the results of randomized controlled trials (RCTs) are strongly preferred to any other means of scientific inquiry when using evidence to support clinical decision making. It is true that findings from RCTs—or better still, a number of RCTs designed to investigate the same issue—are generally rated as the gold standard for determining the cause of a specific condition/outcome (Hedges & Williams, 2014; Melynk-Overholt & Fineholt-Overholt, 2011). Given that participants in RCTs are randomly assigned to an experimental or control group, they are, in fact, the best method for testing the effect of a given variable on an outcome.

For example, an investigator may want to study the effects of a medication designed to diminish anxiety. Individuals with a given level of anxiety are randomly assigned to a group that takes the medication and a group that does not take the medication. After a specified amount of time, anxiety is measured for both groups and a result is determined. The design of the RCT limits a third variable from influencing the outcome—in this case, taking additional medication that could effect anxiety levels (Bench & Metcalfe, 2013).

While results of an RCT are the most dependable outcomes in terms of generalizability to similar settings and populations, they are not the only means to obtain information that can improve practice. Accepting RCTs as the best method for achieving accurate information may be the reason for the concern that EBP will be directed by these studies alone (Mallach & Porter-O'Grady, 2010; Watson, 2012). Realistically, RCTs are not an appropriate design for many study topics. For example, there is some evidence to suggest that infants diagnosed with neonatal abstinence syndrome (babies born to drug-addicted mothers) respond well to darkened, quiet environments (Beauman, 2005). It would not be ethical to withhold that environment in order to further test initial findings. In addition, many activities understood to influence health, such as smoking or running long distances, cannot be studied using an RCT because it would be unethical to randomly assign participants to smoke or run.

Although 30 to 40 projects are ongoing annually in this RFE and an average of 8 to 12 papers are published in peer-reviewed journals yearly, only 3 ongoing projects involve random assignment. In one study, caregivers are examining the influence of a Peanut Ball (a device used to diminish discomfort among women in labor) on a number of variables. Another study is designed to evaluate the difference in two approaches to anesthesia for patients undergoing total knee replacement. The third is designed to evaluate the use of a specific garment for women diagnosed with breast cancer. In each of these studies, participants will be randomized to experimental and control groups.

Numerous practice changes have been instituted locally and nationally from research that did not involve RCTs. The use of a high-risk falls assessment (Corley et al., 2014), an evaluation of nurse preceptor performance (Bradley et al., 2015), and an assessment of deep tissue wound injuries (Honaker, Brockopp, & Moe, 2014) are examples of projects that are not RCTs but have have changed practice locally and nationally.

Another concern regarding EBP is that only findings from quantitative studies constitute evidence. A fear exists that the art of medicine and nursing is lost and that cost of care—not the provision of optimal patient care—is the underlying driving force (Mallach & Porter-O'Grady, 2010; Watson, 2012). For example, there are concerns regarding the value of findings of qualitative studies when compared to quantitative studies. While both of these approaches to scientific inquiry can lead to useful knowledge regarding patient care, two very different philosophies are represented.

While quantitative research seeks to examine what is perceived to be "objective reality," qualitative research is focused on the complexity of a given situation assessed directly in the present. The results of quantitative studies are expressed in numbers, while findings of qualitative studies are expressed in words; as a result, data retrieved from qualitative studies are frequently referred to as "subjective."

A major concern related to the use of qualitative methods is that, unlike the numerical findings of quantitative research, results of qualitative studies are not generalizable to similar settings and populations. A lack of control in qualitative designs, an important component of quantitative research, is another concern. Even so, qualitative research methods frequently produce results that are meaningful in terms of improving clinical practice.

In support of qualitative research, Watson (2012) emphasizes the importance of maintaining a human context as healthcare providers try to find the best evidence for improving patient care. She criticizes traditional methods of inquiry for being mechanistic, closed, and focusing on "parts" as opposed to the "whole." Her concern is that present views of science frequently emphasize disease and/or objectify individuals by ascribing separate categorical variables to them. She speaks of the need to match the method of inquiry to the problem addressed.

For example, an investigator in this RFE designed a qualitative study to examine women's emotional response to the first time they view their mastectomy scars (Davies et al., 2016). There were few data in recent literature to warrant a costly large-sample study. This project provided information that could support further investigation. In addition, comments were sufficiently powerful that changes in care were made at this institution. Publication of study findings in a peer-reviewed journal set the stage for others to design a follow-up examination of this particular patient-care issue.

Gathering Evidence: An Example

A qualitative study in this RFE provided the foundation for a 5-year project culminating in the testing, publication (Corley et al., 2014), and use of the Baptist Health High Risk Falls Assessment (BHHRFA). Findings from interviews of patients as to why they fell added to prior research on inpatient falls. As a result, investigators were able to develop an instrument that could predict falls more consistently than available assessments. The BHHRFA is now used throughout an eight-hospital system as well as other hospitals in the United States.

Evidence-Based Practice: Defining and Achieving: Summary

Clearly, there are many ways to gather evidence that could improve practice. Although scientists have identified levels of evidence in terms of generalizability (see **TABLE 1-1**), meaningful information can still be retrieved from studies that do not

TABLE 1-1 Levels of Evidence

Level of Evidence	Design of Study
1	A randomized controlled trial (experiment) is a study design that removes as many sources of bias as possible from the study process. Participants are allocated to an experimental and control group by chance alone (randomly), one or more interventions are put into place, and the variable of interest is measured.
2	A controlled trial without randomization (quasi-experiment) is a study design that may have greater bias because the experimental and control groups may differ regarding important characteristics.
3	A case control or cohort study is designed to examine existing groups. Data are accessed retrospectively (case control) to compare individuals having a specific condition with those who do not, or two groups of individuals are compared (cohort) over time, with one group having a condition the other does not.

(continues)

TABLE 1-1 Levels of Evidence	*(continued)*
Level of Evidence	**Design of Study**
4	A descriptive study is designed to examine one or more characteristics of a specific group of individuals.
5	A study that uses qualitative methods examines, in considerable depth, a variable of interest within a small group of people. Individuals are purposefully selected based on specific criteria; however, compared to quantitative methods, little control is imposed.

BOX 1-2 Denise McCowan, RN, MSN

Denise, a nurse manager, came to the research office with a concern about the incidence of patient falls on her unit. It appeared that staff were doing what was deemed necessary in the literature to prevent falls, but the incidence was still too high. While there was considerable literature on inpatient falls, there was nothing that described the patients' perspective on why they had fallen. Perhaps patients could shed some light on how to reduce the likelihood of falls or do a better job of predicting falls. She and a research consultant decided to ask nurse supervisors at two hospitals in the same system to interview patients (N=118) as to why they fell within 24 hours after they had fallen. Data retrieved were somewhat different from findings of prior research. For example, some of the patients' concerns were focused on the nurse. They felt nurses were so busy caring for other patients they did not want to bother them for assistance to get out of bed. Data from this qualitative study, along with information retrieved from a comprehensive review of the literature, enabled investigators to design an instrument that could assess patients at high risk for falling. The Baptist Health High Risk Falls Assessment, an instrument that displayed strong sensitivity (ability to predict falls) and specificity (ability to predict those patients who would not fall), was the result of this project.

---

meet a prescribed gold standard. Data that are more subjective than objective can provide information that can lead to additional investigation or changes in practice; the example in **BOX 1-2**, which began with interviews, led to a second project—the development of a useful instrument. Findings from other projects that could be considered subjective can also result in modifications in practice.

▶ Methods Used to Base Practice on Evidence

There are three major hospital-based methods used to develop evidence with a goal of improving clinical practice. EBP projects, quality improvement projects, and research projects use different, but complementary, methods to investigate clinical problems. EBP projects are designed to examine prior evidence concerning a particular clinical issue while incorporating clinical expertise to improve practice. Quality improvement differs from EBP projects and research in that it focuses on how services are delivered. Research uses a formal process to design studies, collect and analyze data of interest, and disseminate findings. Each approach can contribute to obtaining evidence in order to change clinical practice. An important difference, however, is that research, depending on design, can be generalized to similar populations/situations. In addition, there is a greater tendency for research findings to be disseminated through publication and/or presentation, and so findings from research projects are therefore more likely to influence practice across settings.

EBP projects are designed to examine prior evidence concerning a particular clinical issue while incorporating clinical expertise to improve practice. Quality improvement differs from EBP projects and research in that it focuses on how services are delivered. Research uses a formal process to design studies, collect and analyze data of interest, and disseminate findings. Given that the results of research are often publicly disseminated, it is the only strategy that requires investigators to apply for approval from an institutional review board (IRB) prior to initiating research activities. The IRB examines all projects that have the potential for being disseminated locally, regionally, or globally from an ethical point of view. The goal of the IRB is to protect participants' rights and privacy.

While the following sections attempt to describe these strategies as separate entities, it is a mistake to think that clear differentiation is possible. Similarities and differences among the three approaches are described in **TABLE 1-2**. All three approaches

TABLE 1-2 Strategies Used to Access Evidence for Practice

Quality Improvement	EBP Projects	Research
Plan 1. Prepare for change: create team, form goals/theory for change, determine success metrics 2. Investigate possible interventions	1. Pose a clinical question 2. Identify a clinical problem	1. Pose a healthcare-related question 2. Identify a healthcare-related problem
Develop and refine test strategy 1. Conduct small test of proposed change 2. Measure and monitor progress	1. Conduct literature review for best available evidence specific to area of interest	1. Review related literature; involve other disciplines as necessary

(continues)

TABLE 1-2 Strategies Used to Access Evidence for Practice   *(continued)*

Quality Improvement	EBP Projects	Research
Study 1. Analyze initial test results 2. Develop changes to optimize proposed/ongoing change 3. Identify barriers and how to fix 4. Adapt changes to the host organization	1. Critically appraise the evidence	1. Identify research questions and hypotheses
Act 1. Integrate the proposed change on a larger scale 2. Take into consideration the learning process as a small-scale intervention was developing 3. If the proposed change failed, reformulate and reintervene as necessary	1. Combine best evidence with clinical expertise and client (administrator, manager, peers, patients) preferences; Implement change 2. Evaluate the outcomes of the EBP change 3. Share findings	1. Select a theoretical framework or create a conceptual framework 2. Determine appropriate design based upon the research question 3. Describe conceptual framework 4. Identify a target sample/population 5. Design sampling plan 6. Identify target variables to be measured 7. Design sampling plan 8. Adapt the proposed study to align with restrictions of time, budget, participant availability, and materials 9. Obtain IRB approval 10. Implement study and collect data 11. Analyze data 12. Interpret the results 13. Disseminate findings through presentation/publication

to obtaining useful evidence represent clinical scholarship and the shared goal of improving health care (Carter, Mastro, & Vose, 2017).

Evidence-Based Practice Projects

In general, clinicians conducting EBP projects ask clinical questions using a specific format. They access the best evidence available, evaluate that evidence, and integrate it along with clinical expertise. In coming to conclusions regarding changes in practice, patient desires and values are also considered. Practice change outcomes are evaluated and results shared (Melynk, Fineout-Overholt, Stillwell, & Williamson, 2010).

Two models used to guide EBP projects are described below. In general, these projects do not involve data collection and analysis. They are similar to quality improvement efforts in that generalizability of outcomes is not a goal and an IRB application is not a requirement. Individuals pursuing clinical doctorates (DNP) in nursing as opposed to research degrees (PhD) frequently become experts in conducting EBP projects. Often, nurses conducting these projects will develop a clinical question of concern, conduct a comprehensive literature review, critique the evidence found in the review, and make recommendations based on the strength and extent of the findings (Reavy, 2016).

Models Guiding Evidence-Based Practice Projects

Several models guide the design of EBP projects. The Iowa Model of Evidence-Based Practice (Titler et al., 2001) and the Johns Hopkins Nursing Evidence-Based Practice Model (Newhouse, Dearbolt, Poe, Pugh, & White, 2005) are two that are frequently taught in educational programs and used in practice settings. Both of these models are designed to enable changes in practice through examining available evidence related to a clinical problem, but they differ in their approach to considering change: the Iowa Model focuses on piloting potential changes in practice at the bedside, while the Johns Hopkins model provides the steps deemed necessary to efficiently and accurately assess current practices before change is considered.

The Iowa Model of EBP. The Iowa Model of Evidence-Based Practice was developed by Dr. Marita Titler at the University of Iowa Hospital in 1994. This user-friendly model includes a flow chart that helps guide nurses in developing an EBP project and was created to help nurses understand the processes and actions needed to address clinical issues they encounter in practice. The model has four main steps: (1) identify triggering issues/opportunities; (2) assemble, appraise, and synthesize a body of evidence; (3) design and pilot the practice change; and (4) integrate and sustain the practice change. Each step reflects aspects of nursing education, clinical expertise, and the role of the hosting organization/system.

The Iowa Model is well developed and widely used in clinical settings. The model's practical and easily applicable approach is appealing to many nurses. Steps of the model are patient centered and explicit in regard to what needs to be done to reach desired outcomes. The Iowa Model's flow diagram connects multiple bullet points with key reminders intended to notify nurses of factors they may not have addressed, such as taking into account the hosting organization's priorities, identifying key practice stakeholders, and including key personnel to help integrate and sustain recommended practice change.

The Iowa Model was designed to enable evidence-based changes in patient care. Problems that may develop during the recommended process include sufficient evidence is not available to recommend the proposed change in practice, an organization's priorities shift, or the project as designed doesn't justify the proposed change. The model has several "failsafes" or feedback loops should one or more of these problems occur. For example, if sufficient evidence to recommend a practice change is not available, the model guides nurses to conduct additional searches and modify their plan based on new information. Should the organization shift priorities, leaders of the project can modfy their goals accordingly. When results of a project don't warrant a practice change, alternative options are considered and the process of investigation is initiated again.

Although there are some similarities between the Iowa Model and the research process, they differ in a number of ways. Research focuses on systematic inquiry, knowledge development, and dissemination of findings, while the Iowa Model is designed to guide projects that apply to a given setting, and this guidance is not as systematic as guidance provided by the research process. In addition, human subject concerns do not apply, and dissemination of findings is not a goal. Although practice can change dramatically using this process, in general, other institutions do not benefit from the efforts underlying the outcomes.

The Johns Hopkins Nursing Evidence-Based Practice Model. The Johns Hopkins Model was developed by staff members at the Johns Hopkins Hospital in collaboration with faculty at the Johns Hopkins University School of Nursing. This model is designed to incorporate the "best available evidence" into nursing care (Newhouse, Dearbolt, Poe, Pugh, & White, 2005). It is conceptually framed within a triad of concepts from nursing practice: research, education, and practice. Each concept is represented as a corner of a triangle, and each concept is influenced by the other two. The triangle as a whole can be influenced by internal and external factors such as organizational structure/culture, adequate staffing, accreditation agencies, and existing practice standards. Within the triangular model, EBP can be attained by research or nonresearch methods. The focus of the model, however, is not the research or nonresearch methods themselves but rather the process of implementing EBP.

A multidisciplinary approach to use of the model is recommended, and a comprehensive search of the literature is required. An interprofessional team forms a research question following the PICO (problem, intervention, comparison, outcome) format. A practice change is suggested following an intensive review of all evidence. After a change in practice is proposed, the model contains eight steps to create, implement, evaluate, and disseminate the outcomes of the project. Guidelines and tools are available to assist individuals to use the model. Tools designed to help develop meaningful questions and provide criteria for evaluating both research and nonresearch evidence are a component of the model. Unlike the Iowa Model, use of the Johns Hopkins Model is somewhat restricted: It can only be used by signing a copyright agreement. Once the agreement is signed, there are 18 files with guides to assist individuals to use the model.

A submodel is used to help guide nurses during the project process, known as the PET model (Practice question, Evidence, and Translation). Within the PET submodel are 18 steps. These steps are explicit and provide detailed instructions as to how to conduct and implement an EBP project. The Johns Hopkins Model emphasizes interdisciplinary activities. It requires nurses to form a dynamic, testable, and flexible question of interest. Following the development of a question, there is a strong focus on systematically searching, appraising, summarizing, synthesizing, and forming the recommended practice changes based on the synthesis of available evidence.

There are numerous supplemental files and guides provided to aide nurses in conducting a thorough review of the literature before they recommend a change in practice. It is important to clarify that the proposed practice change is not recommended during the formation of the research question but only after thorough collection and appraisal of existing relevant literature have been conducted. The proposed practice change must be based on evidence retrieved from the literature. Following a practice change, there are eight steps to help guide nurses to evaluate and disseminate the results of the project.

Evidence-Based Practice Projects: An Example

Using the Johns Hopkins Model, a comprehensive review of available evidence was conducted on the use of saline during endotracheal suctioning in order to loosen secretions, aid in the expulsion of sputum, and decrease occurrences of ventilator-acquired pneumonia. Following this model, an interdisciplinary team was developed that consisted of critical care nurses and physicians. A comprehensive literature review was conducted, which revealed that saline could harm patients during suctioning. The evidence was reviewed by the team, and changes were implemented; saline was no longer used during suctioning. As a component of this model, patients were followed to ensure the effectiveness of the change in practice.

Quality Improvement

Quality improvement is defined as the efforts of everyone involved in patient care to make changes leading to improved patient outcomes and enhanced learning among healthcare professionals (Batalden & Davidoff, 2007).

Quality Improvement Projects

Within the qualitative improvement process, quality of health care is associated with an organization's service delivery approach. Quality improvement addresses a hospital's systems as they relate to the provision of care by addressing "how things are done." Important components of the process are "when" care is provided, "who" provides care, and "where" it is provided. As such, literature reviews, a necessity when conducting research, may or may not be conducted. Data that reflect patient care services are analyzed in order to show changes in outcomes. Specific patient populations and/or unsatisfactory outcomes, such as delayed length of stay, may be targeted.

Quality improvement activities are most effective when they are individualized to meet a specific organization's needs. For example, insufficient staff able to perform circumcisions on a specific labor and delivery unit may delay timely infant discharge. Prolonging patient hospital stays is inefficient and increases hospital costs. If positive changes in length of stay occur, both improved patient satisfaction and diminished costs may result. While dissemination of the outcomes of quality improvement activities in a given setting may be helpful to other hospital staff, publication of these outcomes is unusual. Unlike research, the goal of these activities is not to generalize to other populations but to resolve problems at a given institution (Health Resources & Services Administration, 2017). As a result, application to an IRB for protections of human subjects is not a requirement.

Quality improvement activities are a component of evaluation in most hospitals. They may provide a foundation for research by identifying a problem that further study could resolve. The falls study, previously described, was a follow-up project based on quality improvement findings. In some instances, research consultants assist quality improvement investigators to analyze data and describe results. For example, a quality improvement coordinator came to the research office with data on patient readmissions within 30 days, and a research consultant helped to analyze the data and write a report for internal dissemination.

Quality Improvement: An Example

The Lean Six Sigma process (George, 2005) is an example of a quality improvement approach frequently used to improve patient care in the hospital setting. This process focuses on eliminating wasted energy and unnecessary practices, improving the efficiency of care delivery, and producing desired patient outcomes. The Six Sigma process targets problematic populations and/or processes specific to a given setting.

The goal of Six Sigma is not to generalize findings but to resolve patient care issues that will lead to greater efficiency and optimal patient care (Health Resources & Services Administration, 2017). For example, a hospital administrator may want to reduce the length of stay among patients with a diagnosis of sepsis by 12 hours. This change could save a hospital millions of dollars over the course of a year. Using the Lean process, a multidisciplinary team is assembled, problems are identified, and potential areas of improvement are determined. These areas of improvement are unique to each unit and their respective hospitals. An important goal of the plan of action is to diminish unnecessary use of valuable resources. The discharge process may be improved by devising clear criteria regarding discharge orders. Earlier discharge would free medical and nursing staff to care for other patients. Using the Lean process, the effects of new discharge criteria would be evaluated over time to ensure that patients regain good health in a timely fashion and are not readmitted to the hospital for the same diagnosis.

The Research Process

Research is "a systematic inquiry that uses disciplined methods to answer questions or solve problems. The ultimate goal of research is to develop, refine, and expand a base of knowledge" (Polit & Beck, 2012, p. 3).

Research Projects

Similar to quality improvement and EBP projects, research conducted in the hospital setting is a process of systematic inquiry aimed toward improving patient care. The research process involves the collection and analysis of pertinent data in order to better understand a specific area of interest. Questions are posed, comprehensive literature reviews are conducted, studies are designed, data are collected and analyzed, and answers to questions are presented (Creswell, 2008; Polit & Hungler, 2016). Findings from quantitative research, depending on design, may be generalized to populations and settings that are similar to those studied. Unlike other processes for investigating clinical problems, research requires a review by an IRB.

While quality improvement and EBP projects are rarely funded, researchers often receive external funding to support their studies. External funding in this RFE of $152,222 (2008–2017) has supported 13 studies. Because federal and state "calls" for funding usually require resources generally found at university medical centers, studies at this institution are funded by vendors or professional organizations. For ethical reasons, all data are analyzed by hospital-based research consultants and outcomes for reports or publications are written by investigators.

Research questions addressed in a hospital setting are not limited in scope and can range from physiological issues—why does general anesthesia have increased side effects among elderly patients?—to psychological concerns—what interventions can diminish preoperative anxiety?—to sociological issues—why do individuals from specific cultures experience pain differently?

Research: An Example

Given appropriate resources and administrative support, nurses can be principal investigators on research projects aimed toward providing optimal patient care. They can also be first authors on submissions to peer-reviewed journals. For example, research that contributed to EBP was conducted in this RFE by an experienced baccalaureate-prepared neonatal intensive care (NICU) nurse. Her study is described in **BOX 1-3**.

Methods Used to Base Practice on Evidence: Summary

EBP projects, quality improvement projects, and research projects are all implemented differently, but each can be helpful in providing meaningful information that leads to practice changes. When individuals with expertise in each of the areas come together, projects can evolve that make a meaningful difference for patients. In this RFE,

> **BOX 1-3** Debra Lewis, RN-NIC, BSN: Effects of Three Nursing Interventions on Thermoregulation in Low-Birthweight Infants
>
> Debra came to the research office with a concern regarding hypothermia among babies on admission to the NICU. She sought advice on testing interventions that would prevent hypothermia in the delivery room. She and the hospital librarian reviewed prior research. With the research consultant, she designed a study to compare three interventions reported as effective in the literature: occlusive wrap, occlusive wrap plus a chemical mattress, and occlusive wrap/chemical mattress plus room-regulated delivery temperatures. The chief nursing officer, the NICU manager, nurse colleagues, and neonatologists supported her efforts. Debra readily learned how to analyze her data to understand the effect of her three interventions. She discovered the probability that positive differences in temperature between each intervention group and her control group would occur (Kruskal-Wallis test). Although the probability that differences occurred was not sufficiently high to be significant, descriptive statistics (means, standard deviations) for each group showed meaningful trends. Debra published her findings (Lewis, Sanders, & Brockopp, 2011); received a national award, in part because of her study; and was asked to be a reviewer for the journal, *Research and Reports in Neonatology*. For her second study on "safe sleep in neonates," she came to the research office with a completed literature review and a clearly delineated research question.

the incidence of patient falls reported to a nurse manager by quality improvement coordinators led to the development of the Baptist Health High Risk Falls Assessment (Corley et al., 2014). Literature reviewed at the unit level as a component of an EBP project resulted in the development of the Honaker Suspected Deep Tissue Injury Severity Scale (Honaker et al., 2014). Quality improvement coordinators, caregivers interested in conducting EBP projects, and clinicians interesting in conducting research can work together to improve practice. Communication among the three areas (EBP, QI [Quality Improvement], and research) is essential so that patients can benefit from the application of these three approaches to obtaining evidence.

▶ Chapter 1 Summary

There are multiple reasons for hospitals to develop an environment that engages clinicians in the research process and provides the support necessary for them to be successful. The move to base practice on evidence is supported by individual practitioners, the federal government, and professional healthcare organizations. Without the active involvement of clinicians at the bedside, not enough research will be conducted to reach the goal of basing 90% of clinical decision making on evidence. Supporting practitioners in their pursuit of optimal patient care can make that goal a reality.

Healthcare delivery has been characterized by increasing cost and delays in incorporating research findings into clinical practice (Muir Gray, 2001). Research conducted in hospital settings by clinicians at the bedside can lead to diminished costs for care and timely implementation of research findings into practice. The study described below impacted practice within a short period of time.

BOX 1-4 Melanie Thompson, RN, ADN: Effect of Music on Preoperative Anxiety

Melanie, a nurse working in the preoperative area of the hospital, was concerned regarding patients' anxiety levels prior to surgery. Working with a research consultant, she designed a study on the effect of music on preoperative anxiety (Thompson, Moe, & Lewis, 2014). Patients (N=137) were assigned to a music or a nonmusic group. Both groups were similar in terms of invasiveness of surgery, gender, initial anxiety level, and age. Participants in the music group listened to instrumental music. Anxiety was assessed using a 0 to 10 visual analogue scale. A score of 0 to 3 was considered to be low anxiety, 4 to 7 moderate anxiety, and 8 to 10 high anxiety. In order to standardize data collection, the primary investigator educated all employees involved in patient care on the unit regarding her study. Her work was responsible for a change in practice within the same year the study was conducted. Her findings—that adults with high levels of anxiety are positively affected by music—prompted the department to offer music to all patients.

With the support of research consultants, clinicians at the bedside in this RFE have conducted studies and published their findings in peer-reviewed journals. As a result of their work, changes in practice have occurred. Since initiating the environment in 2011, 46 articles have been published in peer-reviewed journals. Over the past 4 years, 8 to 10 manuscripts have been accepted for publication annually. The majority of primary investigators and authors of publications are clinicians at the bedside. Two first authors are expert clinicians who hold associate degrees, and 14 are at the baccalaureate level in terms of education.

Reasons why hospital administrators need to engage practitioners in the pursuit of evidence are clear. How to change a culture in order to promote all aspects of EBP is not as clear. While providing resources to assist caregivers to conduct research is an important component of this change process, modifying attitudes may be more important. Caregivers' fears regarding conducting research and beliefs that only individuals with graduate degrees can conduct research and publish findings may need to be addressed. Research consultants can assist with changes in attitudes across the hospital, but administrators need to support this action.

In addition, educators in the hospital setting and in university programs need to prepare new graduates to be actively involved in research activities. Attitude changes regarding the appropriateness of caregivers with undergraduate degrees conducting research could begin in the classroom. Conducting projects with faculty or hospital-based staff could prepare students for their roles post graduation.

Stakeholders in changing the culture would likely include senior administrators, mid-level administrators, educators, and caregivers. Buy-in from each of these groups is most likely necessary if the goal is to modify the culture in an acute care setting. Experience in this RFE suggests that recognition of small successes, even just one publication, is a powerful motivator for others to become interested in participating in research. Affirmation of a caregiver's work by administration has been extremely important in developing and maintaining this RFE.

There are many approaches to developing a hospital environment that promotes caregiver-initiated research. For example, at a nearby hospital, nursing held a symposium that featured caregiver presentations of in-depth literature reviews on a variety of clinical topics. In this RFE, the first research symposium featured the results of several small projects conducted by caregivers. Both approaches were instrumental in moving the institutions toward developing a program of research in order to base practice on evidence, and both events highlighted the importance of EBP and conducting research to obtain evidence. Opening symposia to staff from other institutions can also help to spread awareness of and interest in caregiver-initiated research.

Strategies used to develop this RFE are presented in Chapter 2. Many of these strategies may be productive in other hospital settings. The goal of Chapter 2 is to provide examples of activities that assisted this hospital to develop and maintain an RFE. In addition, the need for as well as the kinds of resources required for an RFE is addressed in Chapter 2. The role of research consultants, the importance of actively supportive administrators, and the need for access to library services and an IRB are presented. Budget issues are included, and the function of a conceptual framework as a basis for practice and consultation is discussed.

References

American Nurses Credentialing Center. (2013). In text reference. *2014 Magnet Application Manual.* Silver Springs, MD.

Baptist Health Lexington. (2014). *Transforming practice through research and publication: 2013–2014. Nursing Report* [Brochure].

Batalden, P., & Davidoff, F. (2007). What is "quality improvement" and how can it transform healthcare? *Quality and Safety in Health Care, 16*(1), 2–3. doi: 10.1136/qshc.2006.022046

Beauman, S. (2005). Identification and management of neonatal abstinence syndrome. *Journal of Infusion Nursing, 28*(3), 159–167.

Bench, S., & Metcalfe, A. (2013) Randomised controlled trials: An introduction for nurse researchers. *Nurse Researcher, 20*(5), 38–44.

Benner, P., Sutphen, M., Leonard, V., & Day, L. (2010). *Educating nurses: A call for radical transformation.* San Fransico, CA: Jossey-Bass.

Bradley, H., Cantrell, D., Dollahan, K., Hall, B., Lewis, P., Merritt, S., . . . , White, D. (2015). Evaluating preceptors: A methodological study. *Journal for Nurses in Professional Development, 31*(3), 164–169. doi:10.1097/NND.0000000000000166

Carter, E., Mastro, K., Vose, C., Rivera, R., & Larson, E. L. (2017). Clarifying the conundrum: Evidence-based practice, quality improvement or research? *Journal of Nursing Administration, 47*(4), 266–270.

Corley, D., Brockopp, D., McCowan, D., Merritt, S., Cobb, T., Johnson, B., Stout, C., . . . , Hall, B. (2014). The Baptist Health high risk falls assessment: A methodological study. *Journal of Nursing Administration, 44*(5), 263–269.

Creswell, J. W. (2008). *Educational research: Planning, conducting, and evaluating quantitative and qualitative research* (3rd ed.). Upper Saddle River, NJ: Pearson.

Davies, C., Brockopp, D., Moe, K., Wheeler, P., Abner, J., & Lengerich, A. (2016). Exploring the lived experience of women immediately following mastectomy: A phenomenological study. *Cancer Nursing, 40*(5), 361–368.

George, M. (2005). *The lean six sigma pocket toolbook.* New York, NY: McGraw-Hill.

Health Resources and Services Administration (2017, February 6). Quality improvement. Retrieved from https://www.hrsa.gov/quality/

Health Resources and Services Administration/Bureau of Health Professions. (2006). What is behind HRSA's projected supply, demand and shortage of registered nurses. Retrieved from https://bhw .hrsa.gov/sites/default/files/bhw/nchwa/projections/nursingprojections.pdf

Hedges, C., & Williams, B. (2014). *Anatomy of research for nurses.* Indianapolis, IN: Sigma Theta Tau International Honor Society of Nursing.

Honaker, J., Brockopp, D., & Moe, K. (2014). Development and Psychometric Testing of the Honaker Suspected Deep Tissue Injury Severity Scale. *Journal of Wound, Ostomy & Continence Nursing, 41*(3), 238–241. doi:10.1097/WON.0000000000000024

Institute of Medicine (2011). *The future of nursing: Leading change, advancing health.* Washington, DC: The National Academies Press.

Jones, S. L., Ashton, C. M., Kiehne, L., Gigliotti, E., Bell-Gordon, C., Disbot, M., . . . , Wray, N. P. (2015). Reductions in sepsis mortality and costs after design and implementation of a nurse-based early recognition and response program. *Joint Commission Journal on Quality and Patient Safety, 41*(11), 483–491.

Kelly, K. P., Turner, A., Gabel, S., McLaughlin, M. K., & Guzetta, C. (2013). National survey of hospital nursing research, part 2: Facilitators and hindrances. *Journal of Nursing Administration, 43*(1), 18–23.

Kjelland, K. Corley, D., Slusher, I., Moe, K., & Brockopp, D. (2014). The best for baby card: An evaluation of factors that influence women's decisions to breastfeed. *Newborn and Infant Nursing Reviews, 14*(1), 23–27.

Malloch, K. & Porter-O'Grady, Y. (2010). *Introduction to evidence based practice in nursing and health care* (2nd ed.). Sudbury, MA: Jones and Bartlett Publishers.

McClelland, N., & Albert, N. (2016). Creating a vision for nursing research by understanding benefits. In N. Albert (Ed.), *Building and sustaining a hospital-based nursing research program.* (Chapter 1, p. 3,4). New York, NY: Springer Publishing Co.

Melynk, B. M., & Fineholt-Overholt, E. (2011). *Evidence-based practice in nursing & healthcare: A guide to best practice.* Philadelphia, PA: Lippincott Williams & Wilkins.

Muir Gray, J. A. (2001). *Evidence-based healthcare* (2nd ed.). Edinburgh, UK: Churchill Livingstone.

Patient Protection and Affordable Care Act, Pub. L. No. 111-148, 124 Stat. 119 [ACA]. (2010). Retrieved from http://www.gpo.gov/fdsys/pkg/PLAW-111publ148/pdf/PLAW-111publ148.pdf

Polit, D. F., & Beck C. T. (2017). *Nursing research: Generating and assessing evidence for nursing practice.* (Page 3). Philadelphia, PA: Wolters Kluwer.

Reavy, K. (2016). *Inquiry and leadership: A resource for the DNP project.* Philadelphia, PA: F.A. Davis Co.

Sackett, D. L., Rosenberg, W. M., Gray, J. A., Haynes, R. B., & Richardson, W. S. (1996) Evidence based medicine: What it is and what it isn't. *British Medical Journal, 312,* 71–72.

Sackett, D., Straus, S., Richardson, W., Rosenberg, W., & Haynes, B. (2000). *Evidence-based medicine.* London, UK: Churchill Livingstone.

Scott, K., McSherry, R. (2008). Evidence-based nursing: Clarifying the concepts for nurses in practice, *Journal of Clinical Nursing* 18, 1085-1095.

Steinbinder, A., & Scherer, E. (2010). Creating nursing system excellence through the forces of Magnetism. In K. Malloch & T. Porter-O'Grady (Eds.), *Introduction to evidence-based practice in nursing and health care.* Sudbury, MA: Jones and Bartlett Publishers.

Tingen, M. S., Burnett, A. H., Murchison, R. B. & Zhu, H. (2009). The importance of nursing research. *Journal of Nursing Education, 48*(3), 167–170.

Thompson, M., Moe, K., & Lewis, P. (2014). The effects of music on diminishing anxiety among preoperative patients. *Journal of Radiology Nursing, 33*(4), 199–202. doi:10.1016/j.jradnu.2014.10 .10.005

Titler, M. G., Kleiber, C., Steelman, V. J., Rakel, B. A., Budreau, G., Everett, L. Q., . . . , Goode, C. J. (2001). The Iowa Model of Evidence-Based Practice to Promote Quality Care. *Critical Care Nursing Clinics of North America, 13*(4), 497–509.

U.S. Bureau of Labor Statistics. (2016). Occupational outlook handbook, 2016 edition. Registered nurses. Retrieved from: http://www.bls.gov/ooh/healthcare/registered-nurses.htm

Watson, Jean. (2012). *Human caring science: A theory of nursing.* Sudbury, MA: Jones and Bartlett Learning.

Wyer, P., Stojanovic, Z., Shaffer, J. A., Placencia, M., Klink, K., Fosina, M. J., . . . , Graham, I. D. (2016). Combining training in knowledge translation with quality improvement reduced 30-day heart failure readmissions in a community hospital: A case study. *Journal of Evaluation in Clinical Practice, 22*(2), 171-179. doi:10.1111/jep.12450

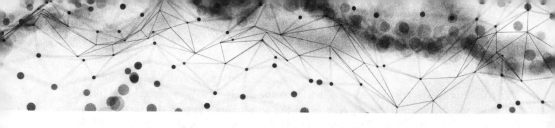

CHAPTER 2

Developing a Research-Friendly Environment: Strategies and Resources

"Leadership is no easy task. It is vital to the success of evidence-based practice processes that the organization be fully committed to establishing evidence as a frame of reference at all levels of doing business."

— **Porter-O'Grady**, 2010

▶ Introduction

This chapter describes strategies and resources that could assist acute care institutions to develop and maintain a hospital environment that supports and encourages research. Based on a successful 10-year experience at a 391-bed Magnet redesignated hospital, this chapter will refer to this hospital and its transition to a research-friendly environment (RFE). Strategies designed to modify negative attitudes toward research are described. Opportunities to reward the success of investigators are identified, and the role of leadership is presented.

Resources necessary to initiate an RFE, as well as resources that can enhance a research program, are detailed. Cost and kind of staff to support research are described. Alternatives to in-house libraries and institutional review boards (IRBs) are also presented. The potential role of a conceptual framework and the importance of supportive leadership are also addressed. Watson's (2008) Theory of Caring is presented as a possible framework that can not only guide nursing practice but also influence the process of consultation within a research office. Watson's theory forms the basis for practice in this RFE.

The kind of leadership necessary to change a traditional hospital culture from one that does not engage in research activities to one that is actively involved is presented. The positive outcomes that occur when the administration provides services such as research consultants, librarians, and IRB coordinators are also described. While 10 years has passed since the development of this RFE, within 3 years, one half-time research consultant was unable to meet the demand for assistance in designing and conducting projects. Presently, 1.5 full-time equivalents (FTEs) staff the research office.

The goal in creating an RFE is to develop a culture that recognizes and rewards questioning, believes in the ability of practitioners to actively participate in research regardless of academic degrees held, and supports the notion that change will be a continuous occurrence in health care. In relation to questioning present practice, nurse managers, nurse educators, chief nursing officers (CNOs), and research consultants can encourage caregivers to feel comfortable bringing their practice concerns forward. An environment that supports questioning is likely to reward creativity and support caregiver autonomy.

For caregivers to actively engage in research, they need to believe they can accomplish their goals. In addition, their colleagues and supervisors need to agree that caregivers at the bedside have the ability to design and conduct studies. A positive attitude toward research throughout the environment can convey the notion that caregivers' clinical experience and ability, rather than degrees held, empower them to pursue goals related to changing practice. Even though caregivers may feel that research is an activity beyond their comfort level, given support and a positive attitude, they are likely to become involved.

Finally, changes will continue to occur within health care. As people live longer, as treatment outcomes improve, and as more surgeries and procedures are performed in an outpatient rather than inpatient setting, changes in the provision of care will continue. Along with changes in patient care comes an increased need for evidence. Caregivers are often the first individuals to experience changes in patients' diagnoses and treatments. As a result, they are ideally suited to identify alternative issues that need to be resolved. Their ideas regarding improving patient care can be evaluated using the research process.

In order to create an RFE in a hospital setting, an assessment of the existing culture, expected outcomes, and available resources may be needed. Modifying a given culture is probably the most difficult task, and also the most important. The culture of an acute care institution can influence both employee satisfaction and patient care. In addition to changing attitudes, opportunities for growth in knowledge and skill are attractive to many caregivers.

Planning for desired outcomes is an effective way to proceed when designing an RFE. For example, nurses understand that the outcome of research in this RFE is publication. What was once a "scary" notion is now an accepted outcome. Nurses are also comfortable with the notion of publication given the support available to them. In terms of support, resources can range from a number of paid individuals to one research consultant with access to a library and an IRB. A designated office, one half-time consultant, a computer, and computer software were sufficient to initiate the RFE at this institution. Administrators' active support and participation in research activities was key to success.

Hospital-based research has a history, even in community hospitals. In many community hospitals across the United States, a modest number of patients are enrolled in clinical trials that are guided by investigators at other institutions. Most of these studies are developed at university medical centers. Apart from these clinical trials, little research is conducted by caregivers at the bedside. This chapter describes the major factors involved in the development of an environment that supports caregivers conducting research at one community hospital.

▶ Conceptual Frameworks

Adopting a conceptual framework to guide practice and set the stage for research activities may be helpful in developing an RFE. While adopting a conceptual framework for clinical practice may not be necessary, a framework can foster curiosity, a desire to learn, and therefore an interest in conducting research. In this RFE, Watson's (2008) Theory of Human Caring was in place prior to the initiation of the research program. The application of this theory, in this setting, had established an environment characterized by a caring response to all individuals. It is possible that this environment played a role in diminishing fear and promoting curiosity sufficient for caregivers to pursue something new and different. Within a caring environment, learning can become a shared goal and the process of conducting research exciting.

The description of the role played by Watson's theory in this RFE is not a recommendation for other settings to adopt this specific view; the purpose of addressing the role her theory plays in this RFE is to describe the benefits that can accrue from setting a conceptual stage for research efforts. There are numerous frameworks that can enable an in-depth examination of patient care and support caregiver-initiated research (George, 2010). Watson's theory is simply one example.

An Example of a Conceptual Framework

Watson's (2008) Theory of Human Caring, adopted at this institution as the foundation for nursing practice, encourages caregivers to examine their practice and look for alternatives. Watson's theory is based on humanistic principles that emphasize kindness to others, development of wholeness in relation to mind and spirit, authenticity, and openness to the unexpected (Watson, 2008). This theory embraces concepts such as taking the initiative, risking failure, working closely with others, and sharing success. Each of these concepts could be applied to the research process: To conduct research, taking initiative is necessary; failing on a first attempt is not unusual; developing a team is productive; and sharing rewards of research activities, such as publication, are essential. Taking initiative—that is, taking the first step to come to the research office—is often the hardest part of the process.

These ideas taken from Watson's theory can assist nurses and other providers to engage in research. Within this framework, employees, as well as patients, are viewed as recipients of caring behaviors, regardless of their roles. Recognition of work well done, celebrations of successes throughout the year, and respect paid to all are incorporated within this framework. The notion of rewarding caregivers for work well done is integral to this theory and has been carried over to research activities.

In addition, these ideas encourage caregivers to try something new and access available resources in order to reach their goals. Given that the greatest challenge when developing an RFE may be changing attitudes toward research in a hospital setting, an openness to new ideas, reflected in this framework, is extremely important. Negative attitudes toward conducting research without a graduate degree, developed in educational programs, can also be a deterrent to engage caregivers in research. In addition, negative attitudes in general can deter nurses from engaging in research activities. For example, anecdotal conversations with new graduate nurses revealed that some faculty teaching research at the undergraduate level in nursing would comment to students at the conclusion of class that they would never have to be involved in research again (Keele, 2011). A desire to consider new ideas, as presented in Watson's theory, might assist nurses to get past that comment and become engaged in research activities.

Originally, Watson's ideas were adopted in relation to nursing practice. They have also played a role in providing a philosophical foundation for the behaviors of research consultants. Acceptance of caregivers' ideas for projects, regardless of knowledge related to the research process, is in keeping with Watson's ideas. Conveying to caregivers that, regardless of their research experience, they can receive support, encouragement, and information that will enable them to be primary investigators and authors also fits with her views. In keeping with her theory, consultants encourage caregivers to conduct research, reward their efforts, and teach them to continue on a research path. Functioning within this framework seems to have helped caregivers to engage in activities outside of their comfort zone. Constructing literature reviews, developing and conducting studies, and publishing findings are new activities to many of the caregivers in this setting.

Conceptual Frameworks: Summary

While a theoretical basis for practice may not be necessary to develop an RFE, all efforts to convey to caregivers that questioning is desirable and supported can move a research program forward. Watson (2012) encourages the development of practice environments that display concern for both patients and caregivers, notions that can support questioning and experimenting with ideas. However, Watson's framework strongly supports qualitative methods of investigation. Most of the projects conducted in this RFE are quantitative in nature. A small percentage are conducted using qualitative methods. Given the predilection for caregivers to conduct quantitative rather than qualitative research, other frameworks that are more traditionally oriented toward the scientific method may be equally or more effective.

▶ The Influence of Leadership

Characteristics shared by successful hospital administrators such as perseverance, continuous interactions with stakeholders, and a need for accountability (Lindsey & Mitchell, 2012) are important to the development of an RFE. Administrators' ongoing active support of a beginning program is essential. In addition, their continuous interaction with caregivers regarding their studies can be viewed as rewarding. A shared vision related to the goal of providing care based on evidence can also move a research program forward.

Accountability for research efforts can be achieved in many ways. At this institution, a record of all interactions between research consultants and caregivers is maintained. This record, the Baptist Health Lexington Grid, describes ongoing activities related to each study. The grid provides a detailed report of consultation activities and an overview of areas of the hospital involved in research. On two occasions, Magnet visitors congratulated the institution for research efforts based on information provided on this grid. An example of the grid is provided in **TABLE 2-1**.

In order to develop an environment that supports research, leaders need to share their concerns regarding patient care; require, whenever possible, that care be based on evidence; act as role models by participating in research activities; and encourage employees to question and learn on a continuous basis. Leaders can also provide financial support for caregivers to present their work at national conferences, develop posters for professional meetings, and pay for individuals to assist with data input.

Administrators play a key role in sharing their concerns relative to patient care. Through sharing their concerns, they can encourage and support the conduct of research. In addition to understanding patient issues, CNOs are usually aware of increasing requirements at all levels of health care to base practice on evidence. In addition, Magnet designation requires nurses at the bedside to be active participants in the research process.

CNOs at Magnet-designated hospitals or those at hospitals seeking designation can role model desired behaviors, set expectations, and acknowledge research activities. At this hospital, the CNO has numerous publications and is editor of an internationally recognized nursing journal. While that kind of involvement is not necessary to develop an RFE, her activities have helped to motivate others to participate in research. Clearly, her support for evidence-based practice (EBP) and research is apparent. Her role modeling of behaviors that encourage caregiver research are an asset to this RFE.

In addition to providing an organizational framework that supports research, leaders can contribute to the development and maintenance of an RFE through their activities and attitudes. In terms of activities, leaders can attend meetings related to research, conduct studies, publish their findings, and/or edit caregivers' submissions. At the practical level, they can provide financial support for data collection and presentation of findings at regional and national conferences. Leaders can role model interest in obtaining evidence for practice and be clear regarding their support of research activities. Acknowledging a caregiver's success can encourage his or her colleagues to become involved in research activities.

Generous Leadership

Acts of generosity by leaders are addressed in the business literature. The phrase "generous leadership" describes activities of administrators that may require spending time and allocating resources that, in most cases, lead to success. Aderson (2012, p. 1) states that "generosity is not primarily about money, and true generosity almost always elicits a generous response." Acts of generosity in developing an RFE at this institution have resulted in approximately eight publications in peer-reviewed journals each year, external funding for 3 to 5 projects annually, and 40 projects ongoing at any time.

Leadership may be the most important component when developing an environment that supports and encourages research. Leaders who believe clinical practice should be based on the best evidence available are essential. Generosity in relation to

TABLE 2-1 The Baptist Health Lexington Grid

Investigators	Study Title	Magnet® Requirements								Nursing and Allied Health Research Office Information								
		Quantitative	Qualitative	Funded	Multisite or Single Site	Assist with IRB	IRB Type	Study Ongoing	Study Complete	Published	Presentation	Developing Idea	Project Design	Measure Selection/Development	Application for Funding	Database Design	Data Analysis	Writing
Allison Fultz, MBA, RT (R) (M) (CT), Melinda Walker, MHA, RT (R)(MR)	Job Satisfaction of Medical Imaging Technologists: A Current Look at Work Environment, Communication and Leadership	✓			S	✓	Exp		✓			✓		✓		✓	✓	✓

Researcher	Project													
Charlie Workman, MS, PT, MBA, CBIS Asst. Dir. Rehab; Karen Craig Ogle, PT, DPT – Director of Rehab Services	Predicting Discharge Destination for Elective Hip and Knee Replacements Using Multidisciplinary Post-Operative Clinical Scoring Tool	✓		S	✓	Exp	✓		✓	L	✓	✓	✓	✓
Andrew Bugajski, RN, BSN, Alex Lengerich, MS, EdS	Effect of eHealth Self-Care Intervention on Symptom Variability, Self-Care Ability, Treatment Adherence and Psychological Distress in a Sample of COPD Patients	✓	✓	S	✓	Exp	✓		✓		✓	✓	✓	

Exp = Experimental

time, resources, and acknowledgment of work well done can encourage caregivers to go above and beyond usual role expectations. In addition to directing caregiver responsibilities and activities, generous leaders spend time facilitating and supporting their employees in terms of their goals.

Generous Leadership: Activities

Leadership activities that support research projects and motivate caregivers to conduct research include providing financial support when necessary, acknowledging all successes, developing an environment that encourages questioning, leading a research group or council, developing and maintaining an avenue for disseminating findings of projects, and supporting educational offerings related to research. A research committee or council led by the CNO can provide considerable support for individuals interested in research.

Modest levels of financial support for research activities can assist in the development and maintenance of an RFE. For the most part, data collection and input are arranged internally and, therefore, investigators do not require financial assistance with those activities. Because travel dollars are limited, research consultants emphasize publication as a means to disseminate findings rather than presentation at conferences.

Acknowledging successes plays an important role in developing and maintaining an RFE. Numerous strategies are used in this RFE to acknowledge success in the research arena: The CNO acknowledges success by email, verbally at department meetings, and/or through meetings with individual caregivers. In Magnet-designated hospitals, successful research projects may be discussed at monthly Magnet Nurse Champion meetings or other clinical nurse gatherings. Publication of manuscripts also reminds caregivers of their success, as does presentation at an annual symposium hosted by the hospital.

Encouraging questioning in a hospital culture may be difficult; however, it is essential to caregivers' willingness to conduct research. Anecdotal data from students completing clinical internships in a variety of regional hospitals suggest that there is a continuum of support at individual institutions regarding questioning of practice. At some clinical sites, questioning practice is welcome, while at others it is not permitted. When administrators at all levels, committee chairs, and bedside staff enjoy questioning and feel comfortable doing so, the number of ongoing projects tends to increase.

In terms of supporting dissemination of findings, research consultants play a major role in assisting caregivers to prepare manuscripts. Writing one on one with caregivers has proved to be productive. In addition to assisting caregivers to write, consultants also sit with caregivers as they submit their manuscripts electronically. In addition, the CNO, nurse managers, and colleagues frequently edit manuscript submissions.

In this RFE, the CNO and the coordinator of the research office cochair a research council. The CNO's presence at each meeting affirms the importance of caregiver-initiated research in this setting. Depending on availability, research council members can include representatives from allied health programs at local universities, including colleges of nursing. In addition, employees of the hospital, such as physical therapists, pharmacists, IRB coordinators, librarians, and consultants from the research office, may join the council. A hospital-based research council usually reviews and approves studies following approval by administration (McClelland & Albertson, 2016). Publications can be presented, research activities described, and ideas for future research activities discussed. This council can serve as a means to publicize the work of the research office and provide support for investigators. Council members may also discuss research activities with their colleagues, encouraging them to become involved.

Educational offerings related to research are limited in this RFE to an hour-long presentation by a research consultant to nurses on the clinical ladder and intermittent offerings to caregivers as requested by administration. The clinical ladder presentation is designed to inform the audience about the opportunities to conduct research within the institution, such as designing a study, joining ongoing studies in some capacity, or completing a brief literature review on a topic of interest.

Nurses may collect data, input data, edit manuscripts, or participate in any other way that teaches them about the research process and assists investigators. The literature review involves obtaining five to seven articles, bullet-pointing important information, making recommendations regarding that information, and presenting a report to a research consultant. Nurses are required to participate in one of those activities for approximately 8 hours in order to sustain their level on the ladder or move to another level.

A workshop for nurse managers on research skills has also been conducted. However, experience in this RFE suggests that caregivers who are interested in conducting research learn research skills best by working with a mentor on a study. Evidence does suggest that a "mentoring" strategy is productive in terms of learning when working with caregivers on research activities (Wallen et al., 2005). Teaching research skills as they apply to a caregiver's study has met with success in terms of investigators continuing to design and conduct projects.

The CNO plays an important role in relation to developing and sustaining a productive research environment. Given that nurses are the largest group of caregivers in hospitals, the CNO is particularly important in encouraging and assisting nurses to engage in research activities. The CNO's verbal support of research activities and EBP, plus a presence at all research functions, can be a powerful force in modifying a culture in the direction of an RFE. The CNO can also be supportive of research by meeting regularly with research consultants. In this RFE, the CNO meets weekly with the coordinator of the research office. These meetings provide administrative support for the coordinator as research office activities are reviewed. In addition, the CNO receives continuous updates related to ongoing research projects.

Professional development can also support the initiation of an RFE. Professional development that includes tuition reimbursement, leadership programs, and continuing education on a number of topics can provide an environment that encourages caregivers to continuously advance their knowledge. A tuition reimbursement program encourages caregivers to return to school and enhance their learning. Permitting research consultants to assist caregivers enrolled in educational programs with required projects is a strategy that helps caregivers be successful in school and may engage their interest in research. In this RFE, students frequently come to the research office for assistance with data input, data analysis, and writing reports.

Nurse leaders other than the CNO can also role model behaviors related to research. Concerns regarding patient care may lead to initiation of research projects, and these nurse leaders can include others on their unit to join a research team. For example, in this RFE, a nurse manager on the neonatal intensive care unit was concerned about the well-being of infants on her unit. She worked with a research consultant to design and conduct a study to determine the effect of sleep surfaces on

BOX 2-1 Regina Stoltz, RN, MSN, APRN: Does the Type of Sleep Surface Influence Infant Well-Being in the NICU?

Regina, manager of the neonatal intensive care unit, was interested in the well-being of the infants on her unit. Because sleep is very important to these tiny infants, she wanted to study the effect of different sleep surfaces on a number of variables. She worked with a research consultant to design a study. The CNO assisted her to obtain external funding from a mattress vendor interested in developing new products. Regina and her team assessed sleep/restfulness, pain, comfort/crying, weight, and vital signs among babies with birthweights <1,700 grams or gestational ages <35 weeks (N=80). Forty infants continued on standard mattresses while 40 were placed on viscoelastic polyurethane mattresses. Differences in variables between mattresses were not significant, though there were clinical findings of importance. Her data suggest that a further examination of the role of sleep surface in the well-being of these infants is warranted. She and her team published her results (Stoltz et al., 2014).

nurses' perceptions of neonates' restfulness, pain, comfort/crying, weight, and vital signs. The CNO, physicians on the unit, and other colleagues supported her efforts. Work time was provided for data collection and meetings to discuss the project. The CNO collaborated with her to identify a funding source for her study and negotiated a contract with a vendor. The study is described in **BOX 2-1**.

Overall, leaders, both administrators and consultants, in this RFE view themselves as facilitators of the success of other individuals. They share a vision of optimal patient care based on evidence, act as role models by participating in and supporting research activities, and help employees at all levels to question and learn on a continuous basis. Generous leadership refers to a willingness among leaders to respect caregivers at all levels of care, value ideas others put forth, and support the actualization of each individual's goals. For example, leaders can initiate and support a nursing model of shared governance. This model enables a change in culture at the grassroots level. Caregivers at the bedside are accustomed to being part of decision making and, as a result, can become leaders and role models in the movement toward basing patient care on evidence. In addition to caregivers at the bedside, nurse managers as well as nurse leaders in other areas can be encouraged to evaluate care on their units and become involved in considering alternatives to present care.

When role modeling of generous leadership begins at the top, a powerful message is sent to employees. For example, CNOs, in addition to meeting with caregivers regarding patient care situations, can also schedule individual performance evaluation meetings with nurses individually. During these meetings, career interests and potential development opportunities can be addressed. Based on the professional goals and aspirations of caregivers, a mutually agreed-upon plan with specified goals and responsibilities can be developed. In relation to nursing, CNOs can nominate nurses for national development programs and encourage them to advance their education with support from the organization or to become involved in research activities. This process at this RFE has resulted in caregivers' writing abstracts for national conference presentations as well as writing for publication.

Another aspect of generous leadership is the willingness of leaders to spend time and energy on developing an RFE. Given that the importance of an event or activity is often associated with a leader's involvement, it may be necessary for the CNO and other leaders to be actively involved, particularly in the beginning stages of development. This commitment of time and interest is a visible and powerful demonstration of the importance of research to the institution.

The Influence of Leadership: Summary

The kind of leadership present in an institution can have a major influence on the development of an RFE. Involvement, support, encouragement, acknowledgment of success, and day-to-day interactions with researchers can lead to increasing caregivers' interest in conducting research. Without the active participation of leaders, resources may not be forthcoming, and the message regarding the importance of EBP may not be conveyed. Without strong and generous support, caregivers' anxiety related to research may remain, and little research activity will occur.

▶ Resources to Support a Research-Friendly Environment

Research consultants, IRB coordinators, and librarians can contribute greatly to the success of an RFE. However, an RFE can begin with one part-time consultant, an association with an IRB at another institution, and access to a medical library, with resources increasing as needed. Assistance with research consultation may be available at local universities. Faculty and doctoral students in nursing and social sciences are individuals who may be interested in assisting caregivers to conduct research on a part-time basis. While it is not necessary to have an on-site IRB and library, having both present facilitates research activities.

As an example, at this institution, the RFE began with one part-time PhD faculty member from a local university. Gradually, the office has grown to include a doctoral fellow (PhD candidate in Counseling Psychology), one PhD-prepared clinical nurse specialist in oncology, and one PhD-prepared physical therapist. Each of the four individuals work approximately 20 hours per week. The faculty member who was the original consultant coordinates all research office activities. The mix of disciplines ensures that many approaches to an idea are considered and encourages caregivers from multiple professions to meet with consultants. Meetings of all consultants as a team occur twice a week to review new and ongoing projects and discuss procedural issues related to studies.

Research Consultants

Having an individual responsible for assisting caregivers to design and conduct research projects available is probably the most important resource when developing an RFE. Personality characteristics of individuals who provide consultation may be as important as their research skills. Jim Collins (2001) concluded in his book, *Good to Great*, that getting the right people on the bus is critical to making and sustaining organizational goals. In the case of developing an RFE, it is important to attract research consultants who bring a respect for the role of caregivers as well as a set of research skills to their role.

Unfortunately, the traditional understanding in health care—that research is conducted by individuals with graduate degrees—can contribute to a reluctance on the part of some individuals prepared at the graduate level to consider becoming research consultants in an acute care practice environment. An understanding that caregivers with little or no preparation in research can conduct meaningful projects is essential to the role of research consultants in this RFE. Relationships are developed on a first-name basis, regardless of consultants' degrees, and characterized by respect for the caregiver's clinical expertise. A sincere interest in the topic in question can also encourage caregivers to engage in research activities.

Malcolm Knowles (1984), an educator who focused on adult learning, believed that adults learn best when teaching is within a context of major interest to the learner. Most caregivers are deeply committed to providing optimal care. Assisting caregivers to address their concerns through conducting research in an area of interest motivates them and their colleagues to learn new skills. When research consultants teach caregivers how to conduct research, they are teaching within the context of the caregivers' study. As caregivers realize that their experience and knowledge at the bedside can be translated into projects that result in practice change, presentations, and publications, they are likely to come to the research office for assistance.

Rather than that of an expert teaching a student, the role of research consultant developed in this RFE involves the concept of collaboration. The notion of shared power, a component of collaboration, can assist nonresearchers in feeling comfortable learning how to conduct research. Caregivers can be viewed as having expertise in clinical areas, while the consultant has expertise in designing and conducting studies. Consultants work with both investigators who have little knowledge of the research process and experienced researchers.

Hospitals designated as Magnet have environments that encourage the exploration of ideas, require the careful tracking of all aspects of care, and expect nurses at the bedside to be actively involved in research activities. Research consultants can assist administrators to develop and maintain an RFE that will meet many Magnet requirements and lead to providing optimal patient care. In this RFE, learning occurs throughout the relationship that develops between consultants and caregivers.

A goal of consultants is to not only assist caregivers to conduct a study but also to prepare them to continue seeking evidence to support their practice. As a result, assessment of caregivers' knowledge related to the research process continues throughout the duration of a study. Some caregivers may understand how to conduct a literature review but not how to analyze data. Others may write well but are not skilled at formulating a research question. Once a productive relationship is established, learning can take place at any phase of the research process. Consultants can be mentors who have an ongoing positive relationship with caregivers (Black, Bungay, Mackay, Balneaves, & Garossimo, 2016); coaches who help caregivers reach personal goals (Feldman & Lankau, 2005); and, of course, teachers.

Given the hesitation present among some caregivers to engage in research, Palmer's (1983) early work on creating a space for learning suggests an approach that might diminish concerns. He states "... to study with a teacher who not only speaks but listens, who not only gives answers but asks questions and welcomes our insights, who provides information and theories that do not close doors but open new ones, who encourages students to help each other learn—to study with such a teacher is to know the power of a learning space" (p. 70). The goal of this RFE has been to develop that kind of space. When it exists, caregivers become excited to learn and move forward with their projects.

Dissemination of findings is a goal of this RFE. There is a desire among caregivers to improve practice across institutions through presentation and publication. Because there are limited hospital funds for caregivers to present at conferences, publication is emphasized more than presentation. On occasion, however, a researcher in this RFE will be sponsored by the hospital or a professional organization to present at a state, national, or international conference. For example, a practicing physical therapist in this RFE was invited to present the findings of one of her studies in Shanghai, China, at the World Cancer Congress (Davies et al., 2017).

Unlike traditional academic writing that usually requires a student to provide a written paper to a teacher who will critique and return the paper with comments, in this RFE, research consultants—depending on need—may sit beside investigators to help them write. Consultants may write the first sentence or paragraph to assist the caregiver to begin the process. For a variety of reasons, the idea of publishing a manuscript is anxiety producing for many caregivers. Often, they have not written anything similar to a manuscript and are uncertain as to where to begin. They may not be comfortable with this kind of writing and need someone to help them initiate the process. In addition, their academic programs may not have prepared them to write research reports.

Assistance with both the research process and writing is available in this RFE. For example, two associate degree–prepared nurses who had not received formal training in research or writing for publication have conducted studies and published their results (Hahn et al., 2015; Thompson, Moe, & Lewis, 2014). They were able to reach their goals of conducting studies and publishing their results with the help of research consultants. One of the lead investigators is conducting a second, funded study. The first attempt for caregivers to complete a manuscript is generally challenging; subsequent attempts appear to be much easier. At the conclusion of the study described in **BOX 2-2**, a consultant worked closely with the investigator to assist her to write an article describing her study.

 BOX 2-2 Linda Bragg, RN, MSN: How Do Patients Perceive Hourly Rounding?

Given that little research had been conducted related to Linda's interest in hourly rounding, she worked with a consultant to design a study. She examined whether or not patients (N=486) believed they (1) had experienced hourly rounding, (2) received an explanation of what hourly rounding seeks to accomplish, (3) were assessed and treated for pain if appropriate, and (4) were assessed as to their satisfaction with their care. Results revealed that, overall, patients were largely satisfied with the hourly rounding process. Concerns were conveyed regarding a lack of consistency in nurses' description of potential side effects of medications and explanations of the purpose of hourly rounding. Because Linda had not written for publication before conducting this study, she worked closely with a consultant to draft an article for submission. They met frequently and at times wrote together. The article was accepted for publication with few changes (Bragg et al., 2016).

The Role of the Institutional Review Board (IRB)

Regulatory oversight of research did not come into existence until the 1950s, following World War II. Since that time, federal regulations have rapidly evolved. The IRB in this RFE was established in the early 1990s. At that time, this Board reviewed a few studies a year; currently, this IRB has oversight of 200 or more studies per year.

All review boards are bound by local, state, and federal regulations. The purpose of the IRB is to protect human subjects. It acts as a governing body to ensure that study participants are provided with information that will enable them to make a sound decision regarding participating in a study. This body also ensures that participants' privacy is respected and they will not be subjected to undue harm as a result of their participation. Although the major focus of IRBs is to ensure protection of study participants regarding privacy and harm, this board can also make recommendations related to whether or not the proposed project is meaningful.

Although review processes can differ among institutions regarding the degree of assistance provided to investigators, when guidance is provided for individuals conducting research, caregivers are more likely to engage in research activities. New investigators, often anxious about the IRB application, need support and encouragement. While IRB coordinators can be in the difficult position of telling applicants that their study cannot move forward, they can also work with research consultants to assist applicants with the process and improve the likelihood of approval of their study.

Prior to applying for approval from an IRB, research consultants assist investigators to answer the following questions: What is the investigator's purpose in designing a particular study? Has the investigator formulated a clear research question? Is the conduct of the study feasible? Is appropriate support available? Has the investigator discussed the project with a research consultant? Overall, the process can be a non-threatening learning activity.

Hospital-based IRBs are made up of professionals representing clinical and administrative areas within the hospital. At many institutions, IRB staff review each application and work with investigators to help them gain board approval. There are three levels of application: exempt, expedited, and full review. These levels represent the degree of potential harm inherent in each application. For example, studies related to populations considered to be "vulnerable," such as infants, prisoners, or the elderly, are categorized as full review and are given greater consideration during the application process. A face-to-face meeting between the IRB and the investigator is required.

Given that the goal of research consultants is to encourage nurses and allied health professionals to conduct research and publish their results, access to an IRB is necessary. While some projects do not require IRB approval, documentation of approval is required for submission of manuscripts to many peer-reviewed journals. For those hospitals that do not have an IRB on-site, there are often universities or other organizations in the area that will process applications.

Unfortunately, anecdotal data in this RFE have revealed that some programs at both undergraduate and graduate levels in nursing do not address ethical concerns regarding research. Students may not be apprised of the necessity of applying to an IRB before initiating a study. New graduates, particularly those working in a Magnet-designated institution, may want to become involved in research activities but are not aware of this extremely important component of the research process. In this RFE, if caregivers are not aware of the importance of ethical issues related to conducting research, consultants and IRB coordinators will assist them to understand the process as they design their projects.

Searching the Literature: The Role of Librarians

Caregivers interested in conducting research need to understand what prior studies on their topic have been conducted. In this RFE, searching the literature is required before any project is designed. Caregivers can access the literature on their personal computers or computers at neighboring institutions (hospitals or universities). Some caregivers have the skills to conduct a search, but others need assistance. While a librarian can be enormously helpful to caregivers in finding and reviewing appropriate articles, a librarian on-site is not necessary; if individuals skilled in searching the literature are available to assist with searches, caregivers can move forward with their projects. Wherever the service is provided, it is important that librarians or individuals with search skills assist new researchers without conveying concern regarding their level of expertise. Experienced caregivers may be years away from examining past research or may not have spent time reviewing the literature in their educational programs. Librarians willing to sit with new researchers the first time they search the literature can teach a skill that can be used repeatedly.

If having librarians is an option for a clinical site, they can support EBP and add to the development of an RFE in numerous ways. Orientation of new employees, classes on computer searches, and visits to units when caregivers cannot leave their patient care responsibilities are activities that can support and promote research activities. A librarian who is available to answer questions regarding the literature as they arise can also support the development of research projects. The librarian in this RFE also supports research consultants by searching the literature as needed for ongoing projects.

Other roles for librarians include supporting caregivers pursuing advanced degrees and assisting caregivers to access specific databases. Given the emphasis on EBP in acute care settings, delivery of accurate information within health care is of great importance. If a delivery system is not in place within an institution, state library organizations and/or database vendors can help hospitals develop one. For example, in the state of Kentucky, a selection of electronic databases and resources called the Kentucky Virtual Library (KYVL) is available to hospitals. Working with the KYVL, institutions can obtain access to digital databases at a cost far below what they would pay individually. Many states offer similar products.

Database vendors can also be helpful if there is a particular product that is not offered by the state library organization. Vendors may be able to provide training and support, either electronically or in person. They typically have a number of promotional materials that are readily available to help launch new services. Depending on the need of the institution, they may be able to work with the information technology department or local webmaster to provide a link on the institution's intranet. Access is usually limited to employees.

If hiring a librarian is not an option, a contact person will need to be designated to work with the state library organization, vendors, educators, administrators, students, and the public. In some cases, institutions have an electronic library in place but will fail to provide a support person to manage the collection. Without someone to champion the collection of resources, the print materials may slowly disappear, electronic databases may not be used, and the organization's investment may be lost or underutilized. In contrast, a librarian or designated contact person can maintain a service that is essential if caregivers want to conduct research.

Appointing a nonlibrarian as contact person would require that person to have a working knowledge of electronic databases. In addition, if the goal is to develop an environment that supports research, they would need to welcome research questions, assist with literature searches, and teach individuals how to use databases. They would also need to understand how to use full-text in-house resources, obtain articles not owned by the hospital, store and retrieve available reference materials, and develop a system for checking out and returning items.

One full-time and one part-time librarian support research in this RFE. They serve caregivers, administrators, patients, and/or patients' families and are available to answer questions these individuals may have regarding evidence related to their specific situations. In addition, these librarians provide services for smaller hospitals in the region that do not have a library on-site. At this hospital, in 2007, there were approximately 3,000 searches of the literature using electronic databases. In recent years, that number has reached 30,000 annually. Potential advantages of having an active information delivery system include an increase in the number of caregivers who return to school, greater access to evidence to support patient care, and assistance with journeys to designation as a Magnet hospital or a Pathway to Excellence institution.

Resources Supporting the Research-Friendly Environment: An Example

Resources necessary to develop and maintain an RFE are largely in the area of staffing support. In this RFE, an experienced faculty member at a local college of nursing was hired half-time to begin assisting caregivers to conduct research. As the need for assistance grew, a fellowship was developed to support a doctoral student in either nursing or psychology. In addition, two doctorally prepared clinical staff, one in physical therapy and one in oncology, joined the research office as consultants on a part-time basis. Both of these individuals were interested in promoting and supporting EBP through conducting research. While they have programs of research in their own areas of expertise, they function as consultants in all clinical areas within the research office.

In addition to staffing support for the RFE, salary dollars are allocated in the nursing administrative budget each year for additional ad hoc research assistant support for data entry. An example of annual costs is presented in **TABLE 2-2**.

Other costs include statistical software licensing, funds for travel to present research findings at conferences, and salary dollars for student nurses to assist with data entry if needed. If abstracts are accepted for presentation, the hospital pays for poster development through a professional printing service. In addition, there is a hospital fund of approximately $20,000 annually, provided through human resources, that supports professional meeting attendance. Clinical staff may request up to $400 for a specific meeting.

Additional costs are minimal. Nurses and other caregivers, given management approval, frequently meet with consultants on their breaks. Many caregivers come to the research office on their own time; they are excited about their projects and willing to spend off-duty time working with consultants.

If administrators ask caregivers to come to the hospital for meetings with consultants, they are compensated at their hourly rate. In most cases, caregivers conducting research work with a team. As a result, activities and responsibilities are shared so that minimal time is spent away from the bedside. Research has become such an integral part of the culture of daily work that caregivers, overall, do not see the time dedicated to this activity as a burden but rather as a component of their professional role.

TABLE 2-2 Annual Costs		
Staffing Resource	**Function**	**Annual Cost**
Nurse Consultant (0.6 FTE)	Provides oversight and direction for research office and activities	$50–$80/hr ($78,000–$124,800 annually)
Doctoral Fellow (PhD Student (0.5 FTE)	Collaborates with principal investigators and teams, assists with design and conduct of studies and writing for publication	$35,000–$40,000
Doctorally Prepared Clinical Nurse Specialist and Physical Therapist (2 x 0.5 FTEs)	Collaborate with principal investigators and teams, assist with design and conduct of studies and writing for publication. Mentor doctoral fellow as needed	$90,000 annually for 1.0 FTE (dependent on salaries)
Total annual cost for Research Office staffing		$294,800 (high estimate)

Funding for Research

Federal and state funding is often difficult to obtain for caregivers working in community hospitals. Because resources that support research are usually more extensive and available in university medical centers, federal and state funding is more likely to be awarded to those institutions. However, grants from vendors, foundations, and professional organizations are a means of providing assistance to hospital-based caregivers conducting research. Caregivers and research consultants work together to develop a one- to five-page proposal for funding. When projects are funded, the research office and research team maintain control over all data collected, data analysis, and any written reports. Since 2008, 13 studies have been funded in this RFE. Support ranges from $2,000 to $26,000 (see **TABLE 2-3**).

▶ Chapter Summary

The process of developing an environment that enables hospital-based caregivers to conduct research and publish their findings may vary. Factors such as organizational goals, desire for Magnet designation, stakeholders, and emphasis on EBP may influence the development and maintenance of an RFE. In this hospital setting, emphasizing the positive outcomes that occur when caregivers participate in research has been important in the development of a research program. Congratulating investigators and publicizing practice changes and publications are usual practices in this institution. Retention

TABLE 2-3 Funding for Research Projects, 2008–2017

Year	Funding Source	Amount	Title
2008	American Organization of Nurse Executives	$8,000	The Succession Map: A Pilot Project
2009	UK Got Grants	$19,000	The Psychological Well-Being of Women Pre- and Post Diagnosis of Breast Cancer
2009	Mattress Vendor	$16,600	An Evaluation of the Efficacy of Using an Alternative Sleep Surface in a Neonatal Population
2010	Daisy Foundation	$2,500	An Evaluation of the Cancer Treatment Index
2011	Pharmaceutical Company	$15,000	An Evaluation of an Intervention to Improve Nurses' Management of Patients' Pain
2011	Supply Vendor	$26,000	An Examination of the Effects of Non-contact Low Frequency Ultrasound on Healing of Suspected Deep Tissue Injuries: A Prospective Study
2013	Association of Nurses in Professional Development	$2,000	Evaluating Preceptors: A Methodological Study
2013	Pharmaceutical Company	$5,000	Education Grant to Support Symposium 2013, "Transforming Practice Through Evidence"
2013	Supply Company	$13,000	An Assessment of a Catheter Cleansing Agent
2014	Baptist Health Lexington Oncology Pathway	$4,634	Preparing Patients for Their New Body Image Following Mastectomy: A Descriptive Qualitative Study
2014	Pharmaceutical Company	$2,200	Wellness Project: MS Population
2016	Supply Vendor	$5,000	The Effect of Essential Oils on Anxiety Among Radiation Oncology Patients

Year	Funding Source	Amount	Title
2017	Supply Vendor	$4,288	Comparison of Post-operative Brassiere and Drain Securement in Women Undergoing Mastectomy With and Without Immediate Reconstruction
2017	Baptist Health Lexington Auxiliary Board	$14,000	The Effect of a Parent Empowerment Program on Length of Stay in the Neonatal ICU
2017	Baptist Health Lexington Foundation	$5,000	The Effect of Hydro Therapy on Well-Being of Neonatal Abstinence Syndrome Infants

of caregivers and improving patient care are shared goals within the RFE. Anecdotal information suggests that nurses, in particular, are proud to work in an environment that supports their intellectual growth by providing multiple learning opportunities.

Organizational goals that include providing EBP and retaining caregivers by making opportunities for growth and learning available are reflected in Magnet criteria for designation. As administrators adopt these goals, caregiver-initiated research is likely to increase. An added outcome is an increasing number of caregivers returning to school to advance their education. Also, the process of evaluation becomes important to bedside caregivers.

Stakeholders across hospitals can play a major role in supporting research activities. Nurses and allied health professionals who want to provide optimal care and advance their knowledge can meet their goals by conducting and publishing research. For caregivers who want to apply to institutions for advanced degrees, publications can set them apart as desirable candidates. Doctoral fellows who work in the research office average five to six publications as coauthor per year.

The extent of interest in EBP may also impact the development of a research program. Given the requirement for physicians to base 90% of their practice on evidence by 2020 (Malloch & O'Grady, 2010), it would seem productive to develop a hospital environment that supports research. The educational preparation of nurses is a major concern related to developing an RFE. In order to engage in research activities, new graduates need basic research skills. Without these skills, they may have difficulty transitioning from school to clinical practice in an acute care Magnet-designated setting.

Strategies used in this RFE to support research include the use of Watson's (2008) Theory of Caring within the research office, involving leaders at all levels in research activities, and providing effective resources to assist caregivers to conduct studies and publish their findings. Resources needed to develop an environment that supports caregivers' involvement in research are modest compared to potential outcomes, which can include positive changes in practice, retention of caregivers, and Magnet designation. In addition to making practice changes on-site, findings of studies can be disseminated through publication, extending practice improvements to other hospital settings.

References

Aderson, E. (2012, July 30). Generous leaders aren't naive: They're confident. *Forbes Magazine.* (Page 1).

Black, A. T., Bungay, V., & Mackay, M. (2016). Understanding mentorship in a research training program for point-of-care clinicians. *Journal of Nursing Administration, 46*(9):444–448.

Bragg, L., Bugajski, A., Marchese, M., Caldwell, R., Houle, L., Thompson, R., , . , Lengerich, A. (2016). How do patients perceive hourly rounding? *Nursing Management, 47*(11), 11–13.

Collins, J. (2001). *Good to great: Why some companies make the leap and others don't.* New York, NY: Harper Business Publishers.

Davies, C. D., Brockopp, D., Moe, K., Wheeler, P., Abner, J., & Lengerich, A. (2016). Exploring the lived experience of women immediately following mastectomy. *Cancer Nursing, 40*(5), 362-368.

Feldman, D. C., & Lankau, M.J. (2005). Executive coaching: A review and agenda for future research. *Journal of Management, 31*(6), 829–848.

George, J. (2011). *Nursing theories: The base for professional nursing practice* (6th ed). New York, NY: Pearson International.

Hahn, J., Byrd, R., Lengerich, A., Hench, J. Ford, C. Byrd, S., & Stoltz, R. (2015). Neonatal abstinence syndrome: The experience of infant massage. *Creative Nursing, 22*(1), 45–50. doi:10.1891/1078-4535.22.1.45

Keele, R. (2011). *Nursing research and evidence-based practice.* Sudbury, MA: Jones and Bartlett Publishers.

Knowles, M. (1984). The *adult learner: A neglected species* (3rd ed.). Houston, TX: Gulf Publishing.

Lindsey, S., & Mitchell, J. (2012). Tomorrow's top healthcare leaders: Five qualities of the healthcare leader of the future. *Becker's Hospital Review.*

Malloch, K., & Porter-O'Grady, Y. (2010). *Introduction to evidence based practice in nursing and health care* (2nd ed.). (Chapter 1, p. 3,4). Sudbury, MA: Jones and Bartlett Publishers.

McClelland, N., & Albert, N. (2016). Creating a vision for nursing research by understanding benefits. In N. Albert (Ed.), *Building and sustaining a hospital-based nursing research program.* New York, NY: Springer Publishing Co.

Melton, L., Lengerich, A., Collins, M , Mckcehan, R., Griggs, P., Payton, I., . . . , Bugajski, D. (2017). Evaluation of safety huddles: A multi-site study. *The Healthcare Manager, 36*(3), 282-287.

Palmer, P. J. (1983). *To know as we are known: A spirituality of education.* San Francisco, CA: Harper-Collins.

Stoltz, R., Byrd, R., Hench, A. J., Slone, T., Brockopp, D., & Moe, K. (2014). Does the type of sleep surface influence infant wellbeing in the NICU? *American Journal of Maternal Child Nursing, 39*(6), 363–368.

Thompson, M., Moe, K., & Lewis, P. (2014). The effects of music on diminishing anxiety among preoperative patients. *Journal of Radiology Nursing, 33*(4), 199–202. doi:10.1016/j.jradnu .2014.10.005

Wallen, B., Mitchell, S., Melynk, B., Fineout-Overholt, E., Miller-Davis, C, Yates, J., & Hastings, C. (2010). Implementing evidence-based practice: Effectiveness of a structured multifaceted mentorship programme. *Journal of Advanced Nursing, 66*(12), 2761–2771.

Watson, J. (2008). *Nursing: The philosophy and science of caring* (Rev. ed.). Boulder: University Press of Colorado.

Watson, J. (2012). *Human caring science: A theory of nursing* (2nd ed.). Boulder: University Press of Colorado.

Weng, Y. H., Kuo, K. N., Yang, C. Y., Lo, H. L., Chen, C., & Chiu, Y. W. (2013). Implementation of evidence-based practice across medical, nursing, pharmacological and allied healthcare professionals: A questionnaire survey in nationwide hospital settings. *Implementation Science, 8,* 112.

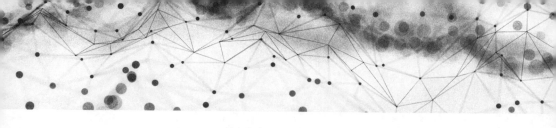

CHAPTER 3

The Research-Friendly Environment Model

"A successful research tradition is one which leads, via its component theories, to the adequate solution of an ever increasing range of empirical and conceptual problems."

— **Watson**, 2012

▶ Introduction

This chapter describes in detail the model developed by the authors as a guide to developing and maintaining an environment that supports and encourages caregivers to conduct research. The Research-Friendly Environment Model (RFEM) has five major components: exploration, formulation, application, analysis, and dissemination. Investigators proceed through each phase as slowly or as quickly as appropriate given their prior research experience or skill level.

The RFEM was developed in response to several years of consultation with caregivers who wanted to conduct research. In developing the model, both the roles and responsibilities of hospital-based caregivers were taken into account. Unlike the traditional academic model, investigators are not required to complete a formal proposal. A comprehensive and detailed process of research consultant/investigator interaction leads to the development of a research question, background for the proposed study, and procedures that will be used. Given a detailed IRB application form used at this institution, investigators can use their IRB application, if desired, to be the guiding document for their study. Using this model, investigators work with consultants through each phase of the model, accessing help as needed. At the conclusion of the model, investigators are prepared to disseminate results internally or externally through presentations or publications. **FIGURE 3-1** shows the model in its entirety. Each phase of the model is also presented and described in detail.

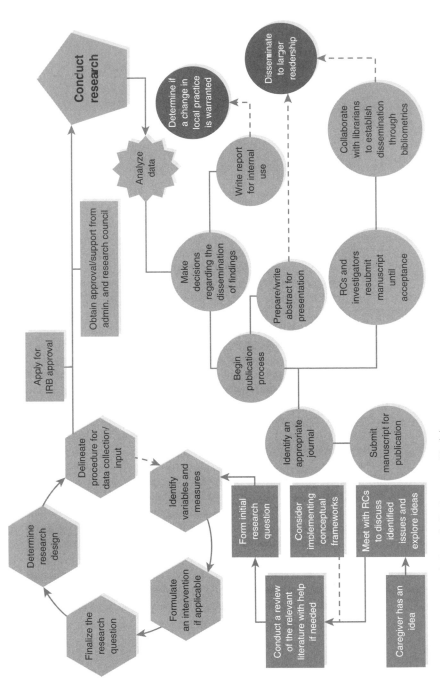

FIGURE 3-1 The Research-Friendly Environment Model.

▶ Exploration

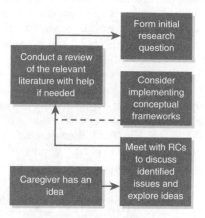

Exploring ideas is the first and most important stage in the RFEM. Using this model, research consultants, administrators, and caregivers who have conducted research encourage their colleagues to bring patient care concerns to research consultants. New investigators are often reluctant to meet with a consultant because they may question or doubt the importance of their idea, whether or not their idea can be translated into a research project, and if they have the skills and/or confidence to conduct research. A major component of the role of consultants is to work with caregivers to help them develop their ideas and begin the process of designing a study. Gradually, as caregivers are met with success, they talk to their colleagues about the opportunities available to assist them to engage in research activities.

Caregiver Has an Idea

The term *caregiver* in the context of this research-friendly environment (RFE) is broadly defined. Those individuals who work toward providing optimal patient care and who interact with patients on a regular basis are considered caregivers within this environment. The ideas investigators bring to the research office are in various stages of clarity and development. In addition, healthcare professionals may express some anxiety as they begin to discuss their idea for a study because they may be concerned that their patient care issues are not important or not researchable. Given this situation, research consultants respect caregivers' ideas and move forward to discuss possible strategies for examining their concerns. Ideas may be put forth as problems ("we have too many falls on our unit") or questions ("What is the level of work satisfaction in my profession?" "What is the effect of massage on infant well-being?"). Examples of problems brought to the research office include increased incidence of Catheter Associated Urinary Tract Infections (CAUTIs), increases in readmissions, inadequate assessment and treatment of deep-tissue wound injuries, anxiety among patients preoperatively, and less than desirable retention of nurses. Questions include "How do women feel when they first look at their mastectomy scars?" "Are caregivers satisfied with the Huddle process?" and "How does music influence cardiac patients to exercise?"

In relation to falls, a nurse manager came to the research office and simply asked, "We have too many patient falls. What can we do?" Through a series of conversations regarding falls and a comprehensive literature review, it became clear that an assessment that could predict falls more effectively than existing assessments was needed to address this patient safety issue. These initial conversations led to a 5-year project to develop an assessment that resulted in a published instrument currently used in a number of hospitals (Corley et al., 2014).

At this institution, falls with injury rates diminished during the period of instrument development. It appears that, in addition to developing a useful high-risk falls assessment, the major focus on falls during that time period helped caregivers to consider fall prevention a priority when giving care. Analyses of data collected revealed factors that contribute to falls, which led to additional projects such as the development of a new toileting protocol. The incidence of falls diminished immediately following the conclusion of the project and continued to be below national benchmarks.

Another example relates to deep-tissue wound injuries. A baccalaureate-prepared nurse came to the office with a concern that patients with these wounds were not doing as well as he thought they could. His initial idea, that treatment with ultrasound could promote healing, led to a funded study assessing the effectiveness of his newly developed ultrasound therapy protocol. In addition to improving practice, the effort resulted in five publications in peer-reviewed journals (Honaker & Forston, 2011; Honaker, Forston, Davis, Weisner, & Morgan, 2013; Honaker, Brockopp, & Moe, 2014a, 2014b; Honaker et al., 2016).

New investigators may come with well-developed formal ideas for a study. For example, a nurse educator came to the office with a desire to develop an instrument that would assess the overall success of nurse preceptor programs. She wanted to evaluate the experience of nurse preceptors, preceptees, and managers of units. She received funding from her professional organization to conduct her study, her project was accepted for presentation nationally in 2016, and she published her instrument (Bradley et al., 2015). As of 2017, she had received twenty-five requests from hospitals across the country to use her assessment. In addition, the preceptorship model at this institution was modified based on the outcomes of her work.

While this nurse educator described her idea in detail, caregivers often come to the research office with general or global ideas. Considerable time can be spent clarifying and delineating an approach to resolving a patient care problem or examining a particular issue. For example, a speech therapist–language pathologist came to the office because she was concerned about the incidence of dysphagia among patients diagnosed with pneumonia. After working with a research consultant, they decided to develop an instrument that could identify patients who would be likely to develop this condition.

In another example, a clinical nurse specialist came to the office with a concern regarding a declining interest among women regarding breastfeeding. She felt that women were not as interested in breastfeeding as they might be if given appropriate interventions and education. With the help of a research consultant she developed the "Best for Baby Card," assessed factors related to decisions to breastfeed, and published her findings (Kjelland, Corley, Slusher, Moe, & Brockopp, 2014). See **BOX 3-1**.

Within the RFEM part of the "discussion of ideas" phase is to provide assistance to the one or more individuals who come to the office to identify other caregivers who could add something to the project and might be interested and willing to participate. If the end goal of the project is publication, identifying coinvestigators at the beginning of the project promotes well-being and high levels of performance among

BOX 3-1 Kim Kjelland, RN, MSN: The Best for Baby Card: An Evaluation of Factors That Influence Women's Decisions to Breastfeed

Kim brought her concern regarding breastfeeding to the research office. She had two questions: Did women understand the benefits of breastfeeding? and What prevented them from making the choice to breastfeed? With assistance from research consultants, she developed a two-phase study. The first phase involved the development and evaluation of the "Best for Baby Card," a pocket-size, laminated card printed with brief statements describing the benefits of breastfeeding. In the second phase, a questionnaire was designed and administered that assessed those factors that influence decisions to breastfeed. Her publication (Kjelland et al., 2014) describes important factors that influence breastfeeding decisions, such as viewing the experience as enjoyable, convenient, and socially acceptable.

team members. Lead investigators can be cautioned to be clear with team members regarding their study responsibilities. Within this model, team members are also told that they will be coauthors on any manuscripts resulting from the project. In terms of writing the manuscript, coauthorship requires either writing components of the manuscript or in-depth editing before submission.

Caregivers' concerns regarding the importance of their research ideas or their ability to conduct research can be a barrier to developing an environment that encourages them to create and conduct studies. Using the RFEM, it has become clear that the process of listening to all aspects of an idea, modifying components of a proposed study in regard to feasibility, and clarifying desired outcomes leads to success. In this RFE, while some ideas for studies have been greatly modified, to date no study or issue has been turned down by consultants as unimportant or not feasible.

Review of Relevant Literature

Investigators can review the literature themselves, ask for help from individuals who have search skills, or work with a librarian if one is available. Research consultants can also assist investigators to search the literature. As the number of investigators grows at an institution, consultants may not have the time to help with searches in addition to providing assistance with design, analysis, and publication. As such, teaching caregivers to perform their own searches can reduce resource needs.

Within this model, before consultants design a study, a literature review is required. Consultants ask investigators to bring or send copies of recent articles that are important to the topic of interest to the research office. They teach investigators who are not familiar with the literature review process how to identify the important components of an article. In order to better understand the literature, investigators, as needed, learn about research design, sample requirements, and statistics. In addition to the investigators' review, one or more consultants read relevant articles and can help investigators to make decisions regarding direction for a study. Consultants are responsible for judging whether the caregivers' review is of sufficient depth to continue the process of designing a study. If depth is insufficient, a librarian or individual with search skills may be asked to assist.

In addition to preparing to design a research project, brief literature reviews (five to seven articles) can be conducted by nurses in fulfillment of a research requirement in hospitals that have nursing clinical ladders or professional advancement models. Nurses who have a particular interest or patient care concern can be guided by consultants to find data-based articles describing studies on their topic. The importance of finding both recent and frequently cited studies is emphasized.

After the search process, caregivers can critique each article and bullet point information related to the problem studied, specific question addressed, literature reviewed, study design, sample, instruments used, and procedures for data collection and analysis. Using this model, caregivers present their written work to consultants and discuss their findings and recommendations. In addition to providing a foundation for a study, reviewing the literature reminds caregivers of the importance of research in moving toward evidence-based practice.

When using the REFM model, studies are not designed until a review of the literature is complete. A formal written review is not necessary; however, bullet points of important information are expected. Through the process of evaluating the literature, caregivers learn the importance of conducting research, improving practice based on available evidence, and the steps of the research process. Hospital employees with experience searching the literature, librarians, research consultants, and clinical experts in specific areas of concern can assist investigators to reach their goals; this support is an important component of the RFEM.

Initial Research Question

The research question is the basic building block for a study. The most important activity in the RFEM is to assist caregivers to develop a research question that is clear and concise. A question such as "What is the well-being of women diagnosed with breast cancer following mastectomy?" or the same idea written as a statement, "This study examines the well-being of women diagnosed with breast cancer following mastectomy," guides the selection of the study design. The discussion that occurs between consultants and caregivers at this point in the model sets the stage for the study. Global ideas need to become specific and measurable. In relation to the thinking process that occurs in these conversations, narrowing the area of interest is likely to be a first step in devising a reasonable research question.

In most cases, caregivers identify an initial question. This question may be modified as variables are specified and measures selected. Examples of initial questions include "What is the effect of a specific sleep surface on the well-being of infants in the NICU setting?" asked by the director of the NICU (Stoltz et al., 2014) or "What is the association between scores on the Baptist Health High Risk Falls Assessment (BHHRFA) and the frequency of falls?" (Corley et al., 2014). Considerable time may be involved in developing a workable question. An example of the process of exploring ideas involving cardiac rehabilitation and exercise is presented in **BOX 3-2**.

Another patient care concern was translated into a feasible study by a wound, ostomy, and continence (WOC) nurse. His research question was "What are the precipitating factors that lead to deep-tissue injuries?" This study, described in **BOX 3-3**, was the first attempt to produce a profile of individuals who experience these injuries.

As an initial idea is discussed, it may become clear that a qualitative rather than quantitative approach may be appropriate. Qualitative research involves an in-depth examination of an issue or problem. The sample is small and data are generally retrieved by interview. For example, a nurse certified in infant massage wanted to examine the effect of teaching infant massage to mothers of babies with neonatal

BOX 3-2 Lindsay Bowles, RN, BSN: The Effect of Music on Mood, Motivation, and Exercise Among Cardiac Rehabilitation Patients

Lindsay, a nurse in the cardiac rehabilitation department, noticed that her patients were noticeably happier and seemed to exercise harder during the holidays, when music was played throughout the facility. She questioned why patients seemed to enjoy exercising more while listening to music. Because cardiac patients need to exercise, Lindsay came to the research office to discuss her idea that music might encourage patients to exercise. After discussing her observations with a consultant, she developed an initial research question: "What is the effect of music on cardiac rehabilitation patients' mood, motivation, and exercise performance?" From her initial question, the remainder of the research process was easily delineated. Lindsay knew from her initial research question that she had to implement music in a structured fashion and develop a way to measure mood, motivation, and exercise performance after patients listened to music. Her initial research question helped her to focus on the tasks at hand and guide her in exploring the most appropriate way to respond to her concern.

BOX 3-3 Jeremy Honaker, RN, BSN, CWOCN: Suspected Deep Tissue Injury Profile: A Pilot Study

Jeremy, a wound ostomy continence (WOC) nurse, was concerned about the incidence and treatment of suspected deep-tissue injuries (DTIs). DTIs represent the early pathogenesis of pressure ulcer development, with a majority of DTIs progressing to stage 3 or 4 pressure ulcers. Little information regarding assessment and/or treatment was available in the literature. He met with a research consultant to discuss his concern. They designed a study to identify factors that could lead to a DTI. He conducted a retrospective chart review of 85 patients who were flagged with suspected DTIs. He discovered that patients who experienced frequent transfers, poor tissue perfusion, surgery, and impaired mobility were most likely to develop a DTI. His study was published (Honaker, Brockopp, & Moe, 2014) and led to additional research in this area.

abstinence syndrome (NAS). NAS babies are born to mothers who are addicted to drugs, and these babies exhibit considerable discomfort for days and often weeks after birth. A research consultant and the investigator determined, through developing the research question and reviewing the literature, that a qualitative approach was most appropriate. Nothing was available in the literature regarding this intervention among these babies. Using qualitative methods, mothers were interviewed, and each conversation was taped. This initial investigation provided an in-depth foundation for further research in addition to changes in practice.

New investigators may want to include too many variables in one study. An understanding of how data are analyzed often helps them focus on the most important issues to investigate. Sample size and availability of participants are other considerations when identifying the number of variables to include in a study. For example, the notion of using multiple *t* tests (i.e., increasing the chance of a type 1 error [finding a significant difference where one does not exist]) may encourage new investigators to rethink the number of variables they want to measure. In one instance, a nurse who wanted to examine anxiety levels pre- and post mastectomy was interested in seven additional variables. Given that her sample would be relatively small (a larger sample would have allowed for a different statistical analysis), she limited her variables to two.

While the literature review may provide interesting information regarding variables related to a given question, as investigators begin to examine how variables can be measured, they might make changes. They could modify their variable selection based on available measures, or they might work with consultants to develop an instrument. Three caregivers within this RFE have developed, tested, and published instruments to fill gaps in the literature; high-risk falls (Corley et al., 2014), preceptor evaluation (Bradley et al., 2015), and deep-tissue injuries (Honaker et al., 2013) have been addressed through rigorous testing.

When working with consultants, forming an initial research question can take 15 minutes or several meetings. In general, new investigators may take longer to think through what they specifically want to accomplish, while experienced investigators tend to have their questions and research design clearly delineated at the initial consultation and seek assistance with other components of the research process.

Exploration: Summary

A welcoming, respectful response to caregivers who come to the research office for assistance may gradually diminish anxiety related to identifying an issue for investigation. At BHLex, this approach is based on the philosophy of caring. Discussion of all aspects of the idea put forward can lead to projects that can change practice locally or across institutions. First-time investigators may work with consultants over several months to arrive at a meaningful, feasible study. Following the first study, they frequently continue working with research consultants to conduct additional research. Experienced researchers often want to meet with consultants to discuss different approaches to analyzing their data.

▶ Formulation

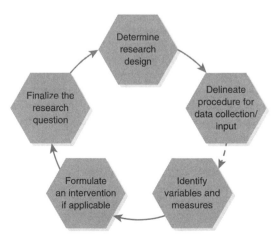

The formulation phase of the model prepares investigators to apply for IRB approval. They identify measures, specify an intervention if applicable, finalize the research question, identify the research design, and describe procedures. At this point, investigators understand prior research on their topic and have narrowed their issue so that a project is feasible. They understand that findings from their study may be useful in changing practice. Measurement is discussed in relation to the model. Chapter 5 presents methods used to develop and test instruments.

Identify Variables and Measures
Variables

A variable, simply put, is something that can be measured and that can vary. As opposed to constants—those things that do not change, such as race—variables may change in terms of quantity or quality, such as the frequency of a diagnosis or the well-being of a group of individuals (Polit, Beck, & Hungler, 2006). New investigators may have difficulty defining their variable of interest. Carefully operationalizing variables—that is, describing how they are defined and measured—is essential to gaining accurate information from the results of a study.

A topic of interest can be identified and defined in multiple ways. For example, the music study described earlier was initiated because, from nurses' perspectives, patients seemed to be happier during their exercise sessions when they listened to music, and so perhaps music would motivate cardiac patients to exercise. The challenge for this research team was to decide what music would be offered and what variables they would measure. The investigators conducted a preliminary survey to discover what kinds of music these patients would like to hear. Questions they addressed regarding the selection of variables included the following: What constitutes happiness? Is mood a construct that should be addressed? What about physiological measures; should they be included? Would music actually impact how long a patient exercised or how hard? Answers, where available, came from the literature. When information was not available in the literature, clinical experts made decisions regarding the variables to consider.

In terms of limiting the number of variables in order to determine a reasonable or feasible sample size, another study, focused on hospital readmissions, was initially designed with too many variables. A nurse wanted to predict the likelihood that adult medical-surgical patients would be readmitted to the hospital within 30 days. He discovered 27 possible predictors (variables) in the literature related to hospital readmission. A research consultant helped him to evaluate the rigor of studies that identified predictors of readmission and, on that basis, he selected those predictors that seemed most likely to occur, reducing the number of variables to 7.

An example of a study in which variables identified from prior research were measured is described in **BOX 3-4**. Two research consultants (doctoral fellows), along with a team of investigators, identified variables in the literature thought to impact nurse retention. They evaluated the rigor of the studies that focused on these variables and selected those that met stringent criteria for research design.

Measures

Selecting an approach to collecting data and identifying a specific instrument are important steps in designing a study. In nursing and the social sciences, face-to-face

BOX 3-4 Drew Bugajski, RN, BSN: The Importance of Factors Related to Nurse Retention: Using the Baptist Health Nurse Retention Questionnaire (BHNRQ)

At the request of hospital administrators, research consultants and a staff nurse designed a two-part study to develop and test an instrument assessing factors related to nurse retention. The team reviewed the literature to identify factors (variables) thought to be important to retaining nurses. Given that little recent research focusing on this issue was available, multiple articles published 10 or more years prior were reviewed. The rigor of studies associated with each variable was assessed, and a list was developed. When the team agreed on variables to be included, a questionnaire was designed. Results demonstrated that each item on the questionnaire was moderately to highly important (Bugajski et al., 2017).

 BOX 3-5 Jeri Hahn, RN, ADN: Neonatal Abstinence Syndrome: The Experience of Infant Massage

Babies born to women who use opioids during pregnancy often experience withdrawal symptoms. These NAS babies frequently experience tremors, difficulty sleeping, poor feeding, yawning, fever, and respiratory distress. Jeri designed an infant massage study to explore the effect of teaching mothers infant massage (Hahn et al., 2016). Mothers would learn to massage their babies and perhaps diminish their symptoms. Participants were interviewed immediately following the education session on massage and 2 weeks post discharge. All participants had continued to massage their infants at the 2-week period. Themes derived from the data included a positive effect on the mother–child relationship, mothers' increased enjoyment of their infants, mothers' sense of empowerment over a difficult situation, and a sense of being able to calm and comfort a child in discomfort.

or telephone interviews are often used in qualitative research, while paper and pencil questionnaires or questionnaires accessed via computers are generally used in quantitative research. Another approach involves simply counting the number of incidents or activities related to the study purpose; for example, in one study guided by this model, Weyl et al. (2014) reported the number of individuals who had colorectal screening over a specified period of time.

Face-to-face interviews are often used when the study topic has not been examined and little is known regarding the area of interest. For example, the neonatal intensive care unit (NICU) nurse who wanted to help mothers cope with the difficulties associated with caring for babies suffering from withdrawal due to their mothers' drug addiction designed a qualitative study and interviewed mothers of these infants. She is a certified infant massage therapist and thought that teaching mothers to massage their infants could help both baby and mother. Her study is described in **BOX 3-5**.

Many investigators in the social or health sciences use paper and pencil questionnaires to measure their variables of interest. Questionnaires may be taken from the literature or developed to meet a specific need. Unfortunately, in some educational settings, students are taught that if they collect data for a study, they must use a rigorously tested, published questionnaire. While that practice is exemplary, there is a need and a place to develop questionnaires and use them without rigorous testing to help investigators answer their questions.

Frequently, issues of interest to caregivers have not been thoroughly addressed in the literature, and tested questionnaires are not available. For example, investigators of five published studies conducted by caregivers at this institution developed questionnaires to collect their data (Kjelland et al., 2014; Lewis, Sanders, & Brockopp, 2011; Melton et al., 2017; Stoltz et al., 2014; Thompson, Moe, & Lewis, 2014). These questionnaires did not undergo rigorous testing, yet they provided useful information regarding caregivers' concerns.

Skills in psychometrics (an area of study that addresses the principles of measurement) are required to design a questionnaire. Items must be carefully articulated and scales to assess content appropriately developed. A recent example of research consultants designing a questionnaire for internal use is related to patient readmissions. At the request of administration, research consultants have taken an interview designed by a national organization regarding patient readmissions and developed items that reflect each component of the interview. This approach will provide numerical data related to several hundred patients rather than themes from a small number of interviewees.

Identify Variables and Measures: Summary

Defining and selecting variables to study, particularly for new investigators, can be a time-consuming task. While caregivers in general, given their practice experience, have exciting ideas for developing studies, they frequently have not thought through the many details regarding the variables of interest that will make their projects successful. The process of an in-depth examination of the variables of interest is an important step toward developing a successful project. Fear of not measuring something in the "right way" can keep caregivers from conducting research. Within this model, consultants convey to caregivers that any area of interest can be measured. Modification of the initial variable of interest may be necessary; however, with modification, measurement is possible. Similarly, there are several methods for collecting data once a measure is developed or selected. To date, face-to-face interviews, phone interviews, paper and pencil questionnaires, and electronic surveys have been used at this RFE to measure specific topics.

Formulate an Intervention if Applicable

Many caregivers want to intervene in some way in order to improve care. While they may have a vision of how they want to change practice, considerable effort is usually necessary to design interventions that are specific, clear, and feasible. Educational offerings, protocols for providing care, and procedures used by caregivers are three categories of interventions often proposed in hospital settings.

For example, using the RFEM as a guide, Schreiber et al. (2012) implemented an educational intervention for nurses in an attempt to improve pain management. The intervention was detailed and replicable. Educational objectives were outlined and directions clearly described so that other investigators would be able to repeat the intervention with a different sample of nurses. Lewis et al. (2011) examined three interventions that can influence thermoregulation of infants in the NICU.

Occlusive wrap alone, occlusive wrap with a chemical mattress, and occlusive wrap plus room-regulated delivery temperatures were evaluated. A consistent temperature protocol was devised. A physical therapist (Davies et al., 2010) evaluated the use of a tool (Astym) to treat scar tissue following mastectomy. In each case, care was taken to make certain that consistency of the intervention was upheld.

For some studies, the intervention is clearly defined; treating deep-tissue injuries with ultrasound (Honaker et al., 2016) is an example of a preset intervention. Many interventions, such as providing music for patients, may differ based on the goal of the study and the patient population. For example, providing music to diminish anxiety among preoperative patients (Thompson, Moe, & Lewis, 2014) is different from making music available to cardiac rehabilitation patients to encourage them to exercise (Bowles, Davies, & Bugajski, 2018). Questions such as the kind of music, length of time patients will listen to music, and whether or not the music option will be ended or modified need to be addressed. For both of these studies, investigators had to clearly describe how music would be available for patients, how it would be delivered, and when it would be available.

Formulate an Intervention: Summary

In studies conducted using the RFEM as a guide, interventions have included massage (Hahn, 2014), ultrasound (Honaker & Forston, 2011; Forston et al., 2013; 2014a; 2014b; 2016), music (Bowles et al., 2018; Thompson et al., 2014), Best for Baby Card (Kjelland et al., 2014), sleep surface (Stoltz et al., 2014), and small group discussions (Lewis et al., 2011). Within this model, when investigators are interested in designing an experiment, quasi-experiment, or qualitative study involving an intervention, research consultants work with them to clearly describe all aspects of the proposed activity. The goal is to provide accurate information at the conclusion of the study and enable caregivers who read the results of these studies to replicate the intervention should they be interested in further examining the same area of interest.

Procedure for Data Collection/Input

Developing a procedure that will guide data collection, data input, and data analysis is a necessary step in the RFEM. Availability of resources and deadlines, if applicable, need to be addressed. Consultants work with investigators to develop a proposed timeline for data collection. Management of their data and preparation of data for input are also outlined. This process is important to the successful completion of a study and also a requirement for IRB approval.

Constructing a timeline relative to collecting data is generally an estimate of the time it will take investigators to collect data. Frequently, data collection takes longer than investigators estimate. Developing as realistic a timeline as possible involves calculating the required number of participants required to meet study goals, gathering information regarding how many participants over a given period of time are available, and judging the likelihood that participants will enroll.

When investigators collect data over a period of months or years, more time than initially estimated is often needed. Changes in the hospital environment can cause difficulties with participant enrollment. For example, investigators trying to enroll women called back for a second mammogram based on initial suspicious results, for a study to assess the psychological well-being of women diagnosed with breast cancer,

BOX 3-6 Judith Schreiber, RN, PhD: Improving Knowledge, Assessment, and Attitudes Related to Pain Management: Evaluation of an Intervention

A group of caregivers interested in the management of pain designed a study to evaluate the influence of an educational intervention on nurses' attitudes and biases. Attendees at a symposium on pain (N=203) were given the Brockopp-Warden Pain Knowledge/Bias Questionnaire immediately after the presentation. Three months after the intervention, 168 nurses responded to the same questionnaire. Differences in nurses' and patients' perceptions of their pain, before and after the intervention, were also collected. Findings revealed that differences in attitudes and biases improved following education; however, similar to findings from prior research, patients with clearly defined physiological problems were more likely to receive effective management of their pain (Schreiber et al., 2014).

had to extend their timeline by several months. Because new equipment was purchased during the data collection period that identified many more callbacks yielding fewer diagnoses, the timeline for data collection was extended. The study was completed and submitted for publication (Lengerich et al., 2018).

Data collection can be simplified if at least one component of the collection process occurs on one occasion. For example, investigators conducting a study on pain management were able to collect initial data at an educational session designed to assist nurses to improve their management of pain (see **BOX 3-6**).

Successfully completing data collection can be a challenge; however, when a clear plan is constructed beforehand, the chance of success increases. Attracting participants; keeping them interested, particularly if more than one data collection point is involved; and ensuring privacy are key components of an effective plan. Understanding the potential value of a given area of interest to potential participants can help attract individuals to the study. For example, a nurse retention study conducted using this model was of great interest to nurses given their commitment to their profession and their dependency on present positions in the hospital (Bugajski et al., 2017). In addition, leaders within the institution, given their concerns regarding nurse retention, supported the project and encouraged nurses to participate. Care was taken, however, to ensure participants' privacy. Negative comments could not be shared with administrators for fear of reprisal. Employees need to be a protected class in terms of research, as their honesty could jeopardize their positions if discovered by administration. In all cases, ensuring that steps are taken to protect the privacy of participants is required by IRB, and, without that assurance, an application will not be approved.

Attending to details related to data collection is extremely important for both the success of the project and receiving IRB approval. For example, hard copy data need to be kept, typically in a locked container behind a locked door. Access to any kind of data needs to be clearly defined. Processes for maintaining participant confidentiality need to be clearly outlined for both hard copy and electronic data. Typically, research consultants and investigators discuss strategies for maintaining participant confidentiality.

Keeping participants involved in an ongoing project can be difficult. Providing participants with an incentive can help. Investigators of a breast cancer study (Davies et al., 2010) needed 38 women diagnosed with breast cancer to respond to a question-naire packet on two different occasions. Because it was a funded study, investigators were able to give participants a gift card following their second response to the packet. In this case, a financial reward was used to encourage participants to remain involved in the study. Providing a modest ($1 to $10) financial reward for completing ques-tionnaires has been shown to increase participation (Dillman, Smyth, & Christian, 2009). Gift cards are easy to manage and readily available.

Data input within this model is facilitated by research consultants. Given that most caregivers in a hospital setting have full-time positions, they need assistance with many aspects of the research process. In addition, few caregivers in this RFE have expertise in designing databases. For these reasons, research consultants construct databases and teach individuals how to input data. When studies are funded, students and/or employees who want to add to their income may be interested in working with data. If funding is not available, possibilities include nurses on a clinical ladder, one or more members of the team of investigators, or a staff member associated with the principal investigator.

Formulation: Summary

A well-defined procedure is key to the success of research projects. However, keep in mind that problems can occur, even though considerable time has been allotted to developing and following a detailed plan. Using this model, research consultants are available to problem solve and redirect data collection activities when necessary. Support from administrators, including the chief nursing officer (CNO), can also assist researchers to resolve any issues that may arise.

▶ Application

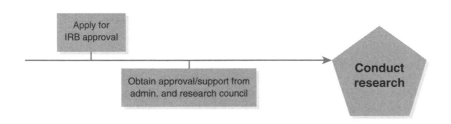

Approval of a proposed study by immediate supervisors; administrators over the area of interest; the CNO; and a research council, if available, is recommended by this model. Problems can be diminished if, prior to submission to the IRB for approval, each stakeholder is provided with the details of the study. Informing colleagues and any interested individuals is also encouraged—the more support generated for a study, the greater the likelihood of success. Investigators are advised to provide the research question, study design, sample of interest plus sample size, measures, and plans for data collection to administrators. Administrators can also make decisions as to the relevance of the proposed project in relation to hospital goals and mission.

In addition, approval processes can often result in improvements in the study design. Reviewers of a proposal can make recommendations that will assist caregivers to conduct meaningful research. For example, members of research councils may have suggestions that will help investigators with data collection. They may be aware of nurses on the clinical ladder who need to be involved in research or students who want to learn more about the research process. Immediate supervisors, once aware of the topic being addressed, can also make helpful suggestions regarding study design and procedures for data collection.

Institutional Review Board Approval

Protecting human subjects and ensuring studies are not harmful to participants are the roles of the IRB. Investigators need to show respect for participants in their studies, describe benefits that can accrue because of the study, and provide "just" treatment of individuals who agree to participate in their research. Applications for IRB approval are similar in requirements across settings. Investigators are asked for the title of the study, contact information for all investigators, administrative approval for the study, location of the study, population of interest, description of intervention, rationale for designing the study, purpose of the study, sample size, recruitment activities, consent process, and a procedure for collecting data that includes the names of those individuals who will have access to the data. All individuals who have access to data must complete a course related to human subjects' rights.

In order for caregivers to gain approval from the IRB, they must engage participants in a consent process. There are multiple types of consent, and the type required for each study is influenced by the kind of information an investigator wants to collect as well as the relative risks to the participants. For low-risk studies that do not require the collection of potentially sensitive information, consent may not be needed; for studies that have minimal risks or collect potentially sensitive information, an implied consent may be needed; and for studies that have higher risks to the participants, where sensitive information is being collected, a full, signed consent needs to be obtained from each participant. Examples of consent forms—if needed—are available through IRBs or research consultants.

Using the RFEM, research consultants work with caregivers to delineate each of the above requirements. They can suggest to caregivers what kind of IRB approval is appropriate and help them with all aspects of research design and procedure. At the conclusion of this process, investigators are prepared to explain their study to their colleagues and supervisors. The IRB office makes all final decisions; however, research consultants often ask for a meeting with an IRB consultant to help make decisions regarding the appropriateness of research activities and the kind of approval necessary for a given study.

Application: Summary

The IRB makes the final decision regarding IRB approval. A positive, helpful attitude among IRB personnel can be an advantage for new investigators. In this RFE, IRB coordinators spend considerable time and effort with investigators in an effort to assist them with issues related to submission and approval. They do, however, expect investigators to work with research consultants to develop clear research questions and an appropriate design for their studies before engaging their office.

▶ Analysis

Given that most caregivers do not routinely work with statistics, they may not feel comfortable analyzing their data without assistance. Some investigators may have initial ideas regarding data analysis, but in general they are likely to want assistance before completing this task. Unfortunately, there is also some anxiety regarding the application of statistics. This chapter provides an overview of the role of research consultants relative to data analysis.

Basic ideas that consultants introduce or reaffirm with investigators include the difference between content analysis for themes and statistical analysis, when and how to use descriptive and inferential statistics, and the meaning and importance of statistical significance. Ensuring that investigators clearly understand the analysis of their data is an important component of the RFEM. As investigators reach the point of writing a manuscript for publication, they need to understand how their data were analyzed if they are to write a meaningful discussion section. Anecdotal data related to research consultants' reviews of journal submissions suggest that authors who do not understand the statistical analysis of their data are unlikely to write a clear results section for their articles. Confusion in this area frequently leads to rejection of a manuscript submission.

Content Analysis

Content analysis is an approach used to analyze words in order to identify meaningful ideas, phrases, or themes. Words, phrases, and/or sentences can convey important information regarding a particular idea. Although content analysis is frequently associated with qualitative research, open-ended questions or a request for comments may be added to the end of numerically scored questionnaires. For example, the study described in **BOX 3-7** was designed to examine job satisfaction among medical technologists. The investigator-designed questionnaire included a section asking participants to comment on their satisfaction with their jobs. This section followed questions requiring a numerical response.

While there are a number of methods for conducting content analysis in the literature (Polit & Beck, 2006), commonalities exist across methods. The process suggested in this model requires investigators to recruit three to five experts to independently review the data. Each expert reads the material several times until an in-depth understanding of content is reached. These experts identify ideas, comments, and/or phrases that are repeated throughout the content. Once this process is complete, reviewers meet with the principal investigator and discuss findings until consensus is reached regarding the identification and relative importance of ideas. Investigators of approximately 20% of studies conducted in this RFE use content analysis as an analysis strategy.

BOX 3-7 Allison Fultz, MBA, RT, and Melinda Walker, MHA, RT: Job Satisfaction of Medical Imaging Technologists: A Current Look at Work Environment, Communication, and Leadership

Two medical imaging managers came to the research office with an interest in assessing job satisfaction within their discipline. They wanted to examine work environment, communication, and leadership. Consultants assisted them to design a questionnaire based on their perceptions of the work situation and the limited literature available on the topic. Numerical results showed differences in satisfaction related to level of experience but no difference based on educational preparation. In addition to asking participants to respond to the closed-ended questions, they were asked to make comments. Those comments revealed three major ideas: a strong desire for competent management/leadership, for effective communication at all levels, and for recognition of staff for good work. The investigators published their findings (Fultz, Walker, Lengerich, & Bugajski, 2017) and presented their study at the hospital's annual symposium.

 BOX 3-8 Claire Davies, PT, PhD: Astym® Therapy Improves Function and Range of Motion Following Mastectomy

Claire, a physical therapist, works with women following mastectomy to improve functioning following surgery to the greatest extent possible. Astym treatment is a handheld instrument applied topically to treat underlying soft tissue damage. Using five measures related to physical functioning, 40 women were assessed both prior to treatment with Astym treatment and posttreatment (discharge). Astym treatment was found to be helpful in relation to physical functioning (Davies, Brockopp, & Moe, 2016). Using descriptive statistics, the sample was described as follows: age range 33 to 75 years, mean age 52 years (SD 11.4). In the results section, mean time to referral for treatment was reported as 7.7 months (SD 13.5) and mean number of treatments completed as 6.7 with an SD of 1.8.

Statistical Analysis: Descriptive

Descriptive statistics are frequently used to reflect the demographics of a sample and may also be used to analyze study results. Means, medians, modes, standard deviations, and frequencies are often used to describe socioeconomic variables such as age, gender, socioeconomic status, and/or educational level of participants. For example, one of the research consultants studied the use of Astym therapy on function and range of motion following mastectomy and described her sample's age, time between mastectomy and treatment with Astym, and number of treatments using means (the average, M) and standard deviations (the average distance from the mean, SD). See **BOX 3-8**.

Statistical Analysis: Inferential Statistics

Inferential statistics can assist investigators to generalize findings from a sample taken from a specific population to other populations. Populations studied guided by this model include infants, pregnant women, mothers of babies withdrawing from opioids, nurses, medical imaging technologists, adult medical-surgical patients, psychiatric patients, patients with pneumonia, and women diagnosed with breast cancer following mastectomy. In each of these studies, whether or not findings could be generalized to other settings is discussed in manuscripts submitted for publication.

In order to most effectively represent a population with a particular sample, participants should be selected using a random selection process. In the case of an experiment, participants in the experimental and control groups should be randomly assigned. Unfortunately, due to resource limitations and time constraints, many studies are conducted using convenience samples. These samples are readily available and not randomly selected. The certainty of generalizing findings to the larger population is, therefore, limited; however, that does not mean that the information gained is not useful.

In experiments—studies where an intervention is evaluated—investigators identify a hypothesis. In the Astym quasi-experimental study described in Box 3-8, the investigator's hypothesis was that Astym would improve physical functioning among women following mastectomy. While the analysis showed the likelihood that using Astym in a larger population would improve functioning, this study was a "before and after" study of one group of patients; random selection did not occur, and there was no control group. Given that design, generalizations to other populations are not as certain as they would be had an RCT been conducted.

Researchers can only conclude from using inferential statistics how probable it is that a given result would hold true for the larger group that the sample represents. Either 0.05 or 0.01 generally represents that likelihood or probability. A probability value of 0.05 means that 95 times out of 100, results are likely to be the same if calculated on samples that share the same characteristics. Similarly, a probability level of 0.01 means that 99 times out of 100 findings are likely to be the same.

Two possibilities are inherent in inferential statistics: Findings may suggest that the outcome has occurred when it really did not (referred to as a type 1 error) or the outcome occurred and is not identified (referred to as a type 2 error). The term *significance* refers to whether or not the analysis shows that the finding will probably occur in the larger population with a certain percentage change (usually 5% [0.05]) that it is incorrect. Significance does not provide any information regarding the meaning or extent of a given finding. A statistical test used to examine the Astym data could show significance (the finding is likely to occur in the larger population), but if that actual difference is small, the outcome of the study may not be clinically important. Anecdotal information in this RFE suggests that caregivers have been taught that the level of significance is the most important outcome of analyses; research consultants work to teach new investigators that clinical findings may be as, or more, important than level of significance.

Inferential statistics are also used to detect differences and relationships. For example, Schreiber et al. (2014) wanted to understand the difference in knowledge and attitudes regarding pain management among nurses before and after an educational intervention. Thompson and colleagues (2014) examined differences in anxiety before and after listening to music in a preoperative setting. In terms of relationships, a number of investigators have examined relationships between scores on assessments and patient outcomes. For example, the relationship between scores on the BHHRFA and the number of falls at four hospitals was investigated (Moe et al. 2014). In addition, Weyl et al. (2014) examined the relationship between a number of factors and the likelihood that adults would undergo colorectal screening.

Analysis of data, particularly using inferential statistics, is often perceived as more challenging than it needs to be. Given that statistics is often taught in educational programs theoretically rather than practically, new investigators come to the research office with great concerns related to analyzing their data. Walking new investigators through basic statistics that relate directly to their projects helps them to understand that they can successfully perform the necessary tasks to produce the results of their studies.

▶ Dissemination

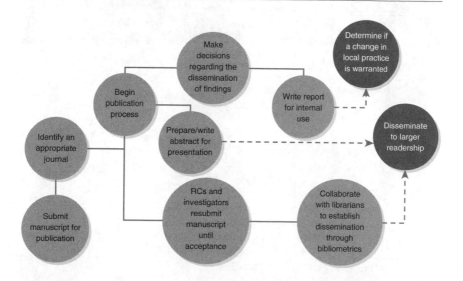

The following is an overview of basic concepts related to disseminating research results. Although publication of results of studies is a major goal of the RFEM, both presentations at local, regional, or national levels and internal reports are included in the model. Discussion of the outcomes of proposed projects occurs early in the planning process. Using the RFEM, consultants assist caregivers to write and submit abstracts, construct internal reports, and develop manuscripts for publication. Depending on the expertise and experience of the caregiver or administrator, consultants work side by side with these individuals. Although not specified in the model, it is strongly suggested that appropriate administrators review all drafts of manuscripts prior to submission. Review of manuscripts by administrators is an accepted practice at this RFE and is delineated in an organizational policy as an expectation.

Delineated in an Organizational Policy Publication

Using this model, 46 manuscripts have been accepted for publication in peer-reviewed journals between 2008 and 2017. In the first year, only one manuscript was published, but this number has gradually increased to an average of eight to ten publications per year (see **TABLE 3-1**). Ninety percent of manuscripts have been accepted on first submission or accepted with minor revisions. Anecdotal data over the years suggest that publication success is related to two major approaches to the publication process: providing encouragement that caregivers have or can learn the skills to conduct research and can write for publication and the specific approach to writing suggested by the RFEM. Given the lack of preparation at the undergraduate level in writing technical reports, caregivers can be concerned about their ability to prepare a manuscript. In these cases, investigators sit with consultants and write together, at least for the first attempt at publication.

TABLE 3-1 Publications Produced from the RFE		
Year	**Citation**	**Professions Involved**
2008	Ross, K., Mathis, S., & Brockopp, D. (2008). Developing a successful palliative care service in an acute care setting. *Journal of Nursing Administration, 38*(6), 282–286. doi:10.1097/01 .NNA.0000312787.88093.ca	Administration Nursing
2010	Davies, C. C., & Brockopp, D. Y. (2010). Use of ASTYM treatment on scar tissue following surgical treatment for breast cancer: A pilot study. *Rehabilitation Oncology, 28*(3), 3–12.	Physical Therapy Nursing
2011	Blair, M., Hill, K. S., Walters, B. J., Senn, L., & Brockopp, D. A. (2011). Caring for nurses: Hospital-based study groups for certification. *Journal of Nurses and Staff Development, 27*(4), 165–169. doi:10.1097/NND.0b013e3181a68aae	Nursing Nursing Administration
	Brockopp, D., Schreiber, J., Hill, K., Altpeter, T., Moe, K., & Merritt, S. (2011). A successful evidence-based practice model in an acute care setting. *Oncology Nursing Forum, 38*(5), 509–511. doi:10.1188/11.onf.509-51	Nursing Psychology Administration
	Honaker, J., & Forston, M. (2011). Adjunctive use of noncontact low-frequency ultrasound for treatment of suspected deep tissue injury: A case series. *Journal of Wound, Ostomy, and Continence Nursing, 38*(4), 394–403. doi:10.1097 /WON.0b013e31821e87eb	Nursing Physical Therapy

Year	Citation	Professions Involved
	Lewis, D. A., Sanders, L. P., & Brockopp, D. Y. (2011). The effect of three nursing interventions on thermoregulation in low birth weight infants. *Neonatal Networks, 30*(3), 160–164. doi:10.1891/0730-0832.30.3.160	Nursing Medicine
2012	Davies, C., & Howell, D. (2012). A qualitative study: Clinical decision making in low back pain. *Physiotherepy Theory and Practice, 28*(2), 95–107. doi:10.3109/09593985.2011.571752	Physical Therapy
	Schreiber, J. A., & Brockopp, D. Y. (2012). Twenty-five years later—what do we know about religion/spirituality and psychological well-being among breast cancer survivors? A systematic review. *Journal of Cancer Survivorship, 6*(1), 82–94. doi:10.1007/s11764-011-0193-7	Nursing
2013	Honaker, J. S., Forston, M. R., Davis, E. A., Wiesner, M. M., & Morgan, J. A. (2013). Effects of non contact low-frequency ultrasound on healing of suspected deep tissue injury: A retrospective analysis. *International Wound Journal, 10*(1), 65–72. doi:10.1111/j.1742-481X.2012.00944.x	Nursing Physical Therapy
	Brockopp, D. Y., Moe, K., Corley, D., & Schreiber, J. (2013). The Baptist Health Lexington evidence-based practice model: A 5-year journey. *Journal of Nursing Administration, 43*(4), 187–193. doi:10.1097/NNA.0b013e31828958e7	Nursing Psychology
	Davies, C., Brockopp, D., & Moe, K. (2013). Internal consistency of the Disability of Arm, Shoulder and Hand (DASH) outcome measure in assessing functional status among breast cancer survivors. *Rehabilitation Oncology, 31*(4), 6–12.	Physical Therapy Nursing Psychology
	Gilbert, P., Rutland, M. D., & Brockopp, D. (2013). Redesigning the work of case management: Testing a predictive model for readmission. *American Journal of Managed Care, 19*(10 Spec No), eS19–eSP25.	Nursing Administration

(continues)

TABLE 3-1 Publications Produced from the RFE		*(continued)*
Year	**Citation**	**Professions Involved**
2014	Schreiber, J. A., Cantrell, D., Moe, K. A., Hench, J., McKinney, E., Preston Lewis, C., . . . , Brockopp, D. (2014). Improving knowledge, assessment, and attitudes related to pain management: Evaluation of an intervention. *Pain Management Nursing, 15*(2), 474–481. doi:10.1016/j.pmn.2012.12.006	Nursing Psychology
	Honaker, J., Brockopp, D., & Moe, K. (2014a). Development and psychometric testing of the Honaker suspected deep tissue injury severity scale. *Journal of Wound, Ostomy, and Continence Nursing, 41*(3), 238–241. doi:10.1097/won.0000000000000024	Nursing Psychology
	Corley, D., Brockopp, D., McCowan, D., Merritt, S., Cobb, T., Johnson, B., . . . , Hall, B. (2014). The Baptist Health High Risk Falls Assessment: A methodological study. *Journal of Nursing Administration, 44*(5), 263–269. doi:10.1097/nna.0000000000000065	Nursing
	Davies, C., Nitz, A. J., Mattacola, C. G., Kitzman, P., Howell, D., Viele, K., . . . , Brockopp, D. (2014). Practice patterns when treating patients with low back pain: A survey of physical therapists. *Physiotherapy Theory and Practice, 30*(6), 399–408. doi:10.3109/09593985.2013.877547	Physical Therapy Nursing
	Honaker, J., Brockopp, D., & Moe, K. (2014b). Suspected deep tissue injury profile: A pilot study. *Advanced Skin and Wound Care, 27*(3), 133–140; quiz 141-132. doi:10.1097/01.asw.0000443267.25288.87	Nursing Psychology
	Kjelland, K., Corley, D., Slusher, I., Moe, K., & Brockopp, D. (2014). The Best for Baby Card: An evaluation of factors that influence women's decisions to breastfeed. *Newborn & Infant Nursing Reviews, 14*(1), 23–27. doi:10.1053/j.nainr.2013.12.007	Nursing Psychology
	Lewis, P. (2014). Knowledge development: Building on a solid foundation. *Clinical Scholars Review for DNP. 7(1),* 48–51.	Nursing

Year	Citation	Professions Involved
	Roser, L. P., Piercy, E. C., & Altpeter, T. (2014). Targeting zero: One hospital's journey to reduce CAUTI. *Nursing Management, 45*(12), 18–20. doi:10.1097/01.NUMA.0000456652.02404.b5	Nursing
	Stoltz, R., Byrd, R., Hench, A. J., Slone, T., Brockopp, D., & Moe, K. (2014). Does the type of sleep surface influence infant wellbeing in the NICU? *American Journal of Maternal Child Nursing, 39*(6), 363–368. doi:10.1097/nmc.0000000000000078	Nursing Psychology
	Thompson, M., Moe, K., & Lewis, C. P. (2014). The effects of music on diminishing anxiety among preoperative patients. *Journal of Radiology Nursing, 33*(4), 199–202. doi:10.1016/j.jradnu.2014.10.005	Nursing Psychology
	Watkins, S., Corley, D., Cleeter, D., Moe, K., & Brockopp, D. (2014). Implementing a nurse leader fellowship model. *Nursing Management, 45*(7), 53–55. doi:10.1097/01.NUMA.0000451038.15082.b7	Nursing Psychology
	Weyl, H., Yackzan, S., Ross, K., Henson, A., Moe, K., & Lewis, C. P. (2015). Understanding colorectal screening behaviors and factors associated with screening in a community hospital setting. *Clinical Journal of Oncology Nursing, 19*(1), 89–93. doi:10.1188/15.cjon.89-93	Nursing Psychology Administration
2015	Alaloul, F., Brockopp, D. Y., Andrykowski, M. A., Hall, L. A., & Al Nusairat, T. S. (2015). Quality of life in Arab Muslim cancer survivors following hematopoietic stem cell transplantation: Comparison with matched healthy group. *Support Care Cancer, 23*(7), 2157–2164. doi:10.1007/s00520-014-2583-7	Nursing Psychology
	Bradley, H., Cantrell, D., Dollahan, K., Hall, B., Lewis, P., Merritt, S., . . . , White, D. (2015). Evaluating preceptors: A methodological study. *Journal of Nurses Professional Development, 31*(3), 164–169. doi:10.1097/nnd.0000000000000166	Nursing

(continues)

	TABLE 3-1 Publications Produced from the RFE	*(continued)*
Year	**Citation**	**Professions Involved**
	Davies, C., Brockopp, D., & Moe, K. (2015). Test-retest and internal consistency of the Disability of Arm, Shoulder and Hand (DASH) outcome measure in assessing functional status among breast cancer survivors with lymphedema. *Rehabilitation Oncology, 33*(1), 28–31.	Physical Therapy Nursing Psychology
	Lewis, C. P., Corley, D. J., Lake, N., Brockopp, D., & Moe, K. (2015). Overcoming barriers to effective pain management: The use of professionally directed small group discussions. *Pain Management Nursing, 16*(2), 121–127. doi:10.1016/j.pmn.2014.05.002	Nursing Psychology
	Moe, K., Brockopp, D., McCowan, D., Merritt, S., & Hall, B. (2015). Major predictors of inpatient falls: A multisite study. *Journal of Nursing Administration, 45*(10), 498–502. doi:10.1097/nna.0000000000000241	Nursing Psychology
	Hahn, J., Byrd, R., Lengerich, A., Hench, J., Ford, C., Byrd, S., Stoltz, R. (2015) Neonatal abstinence syndrome: The experience of infant massage. *Creative Nursing, 22*(1), 45–50. doi:10.1891/1078-4535.22.1.45	Nursing Psychology
2016	Davies, C. C., Brockopp, D., & Moe, K. (2016). Astym therapy improves function and range of motion following mastectomy. *Breast Cancer, 8,* 39–45. doi:10.2147/bctt.s102598	Physical Therapy Nursing Psychology
	Brockopp, D., Hill, K., Moe, K., & Wright, L. (2016). Transforming practice through publication: A community hospital approach to the creation of a research-intensive environment. *Journal of Nursing Administration, 46*(1), 38-42. doi:10.1097/nna.0000000000000294	Nursing Psychology Librarian
	Bugajski, A., Lengerich, A., McCowan, D., Merritt, S., Moe, K., Hall, B., . . . , Brockopp, D. (2017). The Baptist Health High-Risk Falls Assessment: One assessment fits all. *Journal of Nursing Care Quality, 32*(2), 114–119. doi:10.1097/ncq.0000000000000220	Nursing Psychology

Year	Citation	Professions Involved
	Honaker, J. S., Forston, M. R., Davis, E. A., Weisner, M. M., Morgan, J. A., & Sacca, E. (2016). The effect of adjunctive noncontact low frequency ultrasound on deep tissue pressure injury. *Wound Repair and Regeneration, 24*(6), 1081–1088. doi:10.1111/wrr.12479	Nursing Physical Therapy
	Melton, L., Lengerich, A., Collins, M., McKeehan, R., Dunn, D., Griggs, P., . . . , Bugajski, A. (2017). Evaluation of huddles: A multisite study. *Health Care Management, 36*(3), 282–287. doi:10.1097/hcm.0000000000000171	Nursing Psychology
	Bragg, L., Bugajski, A., Marchese, M., Caldwell, R., Houle, L., Thompson, R., . . . , Lengerich, A. (2016). How do patients perceive hourly rounding? *Nursing Management, 47*(11), 11–13. doi:10.1097/01.NUMA.0000502807.60295.c5	Nursing
	Davies, C. C., Colon, G., Geyer, H., Pfalzer, L., & Fisher, M. I. (2016). Oncology EDGE Task Force on Prostate Cancer Outcomes: A systematic review of outcome measures for functional mobility. *Rehabilitation Oncology, 34*(3), 82–96. doi:10.1097/01.REO.0000000000000029	Physical Therapy
2017	Davies, C. C., Brockopp, D., Moe, K., Wheeler, P., Abner, J., & Lengerich, A. (2017). Exploring the lived experience of women immediately following mastectomy: A phenomenological study. *Cancer Nursing, 40*(5), 361–368. doi:10.1097/ncc.0000000000000413	Physical Therapy Nursing Psychology
	Lengerich, A., Bugajski, A., Marchese, M., Hall, B., Yackzan, S., Davies, C., & Brockopp, D. (2017). The Baptist Health Nurse Retention Questionnaire: A methodological study, part 1. *Journal of Nursing Administration, 47*(5), 289–293. doi:10.1097/nna.0000000000000480	Psychology Nursing
	Bugajski, A., Lengerich, A., Marchese, M., Hall, B., Yackzan, S., Davies, C., & Brockopp, D. (2017). The importance of factors related to nurse retention: Using the Baptist Health Nurse Retention Questionnaire, Part 2. *Journal of Nursing Administration, 47*(6), 308–312. doi:10.1097/nna.0000000000000486	Nursing Psychology

(continues)

TABLE 3-1 Publications Produced from the RFE		*(continued)*
Year	**Citation**	**Professions Involved**
	Levenhagen, K., Davies, C., Perdomo, M., Ryans, K., & Gilchrist, L. (2017a). Diagnosis of upper-quadrant lymphedema secondary to cancer: Clinical Practice Guideline From the Oncology Section of APTA. *Rehabilitation Oncology, 35*(3), e1–e18. doi:10.1097/01.reo.0000000000000073	Physical Therapy
	Levenhagen, K., Davies, C., Perdomo, M., Ryans, K., & Gilchrist, L. (2017b). Diagnosis of upper quadrant lymphedema secondary to cancer: Clinical Practice Guideline From the Oncology Section of the American Physical Therapy Association. *Physical Therapy, 97*(7), 729–745. doi:10.1093/ptj/pzx050	Physical Therapy
	Davies, C., Levenhagen, K., Ryans, K., Perdomo, M., & Gilchrist, L. (2017a). An executive summary of the Clinical Practice Guideline: Diagnosis of upper-quadrant lymphedema secondary to cancer. *Rehabilitation Oncology, 35*(3), 114–118. doi:10.1097/01.REO.0000000000000075	Physical Therapy
	Davies, C., Levenhagen, K., Ryans, K., Perdomo, M., & Gilchrist, L. (2017b). How can a clinical practice guideline enhance my practice? *Rehabilitation Oncology, 35*(3), 111–113. doi:10.1097/01.REO.0000000000000076	Physical Therapy
	Davies, C. C., Lengerich, A., Bugajski, A., Brockopp, D. Use of the patient-specific functional scale in patients with breast cancer. Manuscript submitted for publication.	Physical Therapy Psychology Nursing

The initial decision to submit a manuscript for publication is based on whether or not the information retrieved from the results of a study is likely to be of interest to a particular audience. Consultants and investigators work together to make that decision. They try to ensure that prior research in the study area is clearly understood and incorporated in a proposed manuscript. Another important step is to select a journal. Caregivers may think it is sufficient to identify a journal based on content reflecting the study area, but in addition to content focus, consultants and investigators spend considerable time assessing journals for the rigor of design in the studies published, as well as methods and statistics that seem to prevail in a given

> **BOX 3-9** Preston Lewis, RN, MSN, DNP, CCRN: Overcoming Barriers to Effective Pain Management: The Use of Professionally Directed Small Group Discussions
>
> Concerns regarding the management of pain of critically ill patients motivated the investigator to design a quasi-experimental intervention study that could increase nurses' knowledge of pain management and diminish their biases toward specific patient groups. Professionally directed group discussions were held in order to better understand nurses' lack of knowledge and biases as well as promote self-awareness of unknown biases among various patient populations. The discussions included (1) identifying biases with specific patient populations, (2) learning how to effectively acknowledge personal biases while managing pain for critical care patients, and (3) gaining new knowledge regarding evidence-based assessments and interventions to improve overall pain management outcomes. Results of the study demonstrated positive changes in mean knowledge and bias scores toward several patient populations (Lewis et al., 2015). While there are a number of journals focused on the management of pain, this manuscript was about nurses, members of groups were not randomly assigned, and basic statistics were used to analyze data retrieved. After examining these factors, the *Journal of Pain Management Nursing* was selected for submission.

journal. Editors of journals who are largely interested in randomized controlled trials for study design are unlikely to accept descriptive studies for review. The study in **BOX 3-9**, designed to improve pain management among critical care nurses, was submitted and accepted by the *Journal of Pain Management Nursing* after an assessment of possible journals.

Within this model, it is also recommended that two to three individuals who are not involved in a specific study review the article for clarity. Consultants often fill this role. In addition, content experts may be asked to read a manuscript for accuracy of content or suggestions for strengthening the manuscript. The last step in the publication process is one of assisting the investigator to actually submit a manuscript online. Consultants do not perform that task for individuals but sit with them so that learning about the process occurs. When articles are accepted with revisions, consultants discuss approaches to revising the content.

Consultants developed a format that guides responses to critiques in a way that clarifies changes, provides rationale for each change, and ensures that all criticisms have been addressed. A table is constructed with each criticism identified in a column, and a response to each comment is written in the next column with page and line number where change has been made. When a requested change is not made, the rationale for not responding to a particular critique is included along with an appropriate reference.

▶ Chapter Summary

Given potential improvements in practice through conducting research, dissemination of findings conducted is an important component of the RFEM. Caregivers' ideas at

TABLE 3-2 Impact of Baptist Health Lexington's Research Office	
Citations & Access of Publications	**Total Dissemination, 2008–2016**
Total citations in the United States: Based on location of first authors and journals	26 states
Total citations in countries worldwide: Based on location of first authors and journals	30 countries
Total citations in published literature worldwide (journals, books, doctoral and Master's Theses/Projects)	205
Total number of times publications were accessed/downloaded via online libraries internationally	28,580

Note: Data for 2017 publications is not currently available.

one institution can be replicated by others, or changes in practice can be made based on reported outcomes. For example, over the past 10 years, publications in this RFE have been accessed more than 28,580 times (See **TABLE 3-2**).

The RFEM can provide guidance for caregivers who want to conduct research, administrators who want to develop an environment that encourages caregiver-initiated research, and research consultants as they devise plans for helping caregivers conduct studies. The steps in the model have guided research activities in a community hospital for 10 years. The guidance provided has contributed to productivity in terms of numbers of studies conducted, manuscripts accepted for publication, and learning among caregivers regarding research and publication.

References

Alaloul, F., Brockopp, D. Y., Andrykowski, M. A., Hall, L. A., & Al Nusairat, T. S. (2015). Quality of life in Arab Muslim cancer survivors following hematopoietic stem cell transplantation: Comparison with matched healthy group. *Support Care Cancer, 23*(7), 2157–2164. doi:10.1007/s00520-014-2583-7

Blair, M., Hill, K. S., Walters, B. J., Senn, L., & Brockopp, D. A. (2011). Caring for nurses: Hospital-based study groups for certification. *Journal of Nurses and Staff Development, 27*(4), 165–169. doi:10.1097/NND.0b013e3181a68aae

Bowles, L., Curtis, J., Davies, C., Lengerich, A., & Bugajski, A. (2018). Effect of music on mood, motivation and physical exercise in cardiac rehabilitation patients. Manuscript submitted for publication.

Bradley, H., Cantrell, D., Dollahan, K., Hall, B., Lewis, P., Merritt, S., . . . , White, D. (2015). Evaluating preceptors: A methodological study. *Journal of Nurses Professional Development, 31*(3), 164–169. doi:10.1097/nnd.0000000000000166

Bragg, L., Bugajski, A., Marchese, M., Caldwell, R., Houle, L., Thompson, R., . . . , Lengerich, A. (2016). How do patients perceive hourly rounding? *Nursing Management, 47*(11), 11–13. doi:10.1097/01 .NUMA.0000502807.60295.c5

Brockopp, D., Hill, K., Moe, K., & Wright, L. (2016). Transforming practice through publication: A community hospital approach to the creation of a research-intensive environment. *Journal of Nursing Administration, 46*(1), 38–42. doi:10.1097/nna.0000000000000294

Brockopp, D., Schreiber, J., Hill, K., Altpeter, T., Moe, K., & Merritt, S. (2011). A successful evidence-based practice model in an acute care setting. *Oncology Nursing Forum, 38*(5), 509–511. doi:10.1188/11.onf.509-51

Brockopp, D. Y., Moe, K., Corley, D., & Schreiber, J. (2013). The Baptist Health Lexington evidence-based practice model: A 5-year journey. *Journal of Nursing Administration, 43*(4), 187–193. doi:10.1097 /NNA.0b013e31828958e7

Bugajski, A., Lengerich, A., Marchese, M., Hall, B., Yackzan, S., Davies, C., & Brockopp, D. (2017). The importance of factors related to nurse retention: Using the Baptist Health Nurse Retention questionnaire, part 2. *Journal of Nursing Administration, 47*(6), 308–312. doi:10.1097/nna.0000000000000486

Corley, D., Brockopp, D., McCowan, D., Merritt, S., Cobb, T., Johnson, B., . . . , Hall, B. (2014). The Baptist Health high risk falls assessment: A methodological study. *Journal of Nursing Administration, 44*(5), 263–269. doi:10.1097/nna.0000000000000065

Davies, C., Brockopp, D., & Moe, K. (2013). Internal consistency of the disability of arm, shoulder and hand (DASH) outcome measure in assessing functional status among breast cancer survivors. *Rehabilitation Oncology, 31*(4), 6–12.

Davies, C., Brockopp, D., & Moe, K. (2015). Test-retest and internal consistency of the disability of arm, shoulder and hand (DASH) outcome measure in assessing functional status among breast cancer survivors with lymphedema. *Rehabilitation Oncology, 33*(1), 28–31.

Davies, C., & Howell, D. (2012). A qualitative study: Clinical decision making in low back pain. *Physiotherapy Theory and Practice, 28*(2), 95–107. doi:10.3109/09593985.2011.571752

Davies, C., Levenhagen, K., Ryans, K., Perdomo, M., & Gilchrist, L. (2017a). An executive summary of the clinical practice guideline: Diagnosis of upper-quadrant lymphedema secondary to cancer. *Rehabilitation Oncology, 35*(3), 114–118. doi:10.1097/01.REO.0000000000000075

Davies, C., Levenhagen, K., Ryans, K., Perdomo, M., & Gilchrist, L. (2017b). How can a clinical practice guideline enhance my practice? *Rehabilitation Oncology, 35*(3), 111–113. doi:10.1097/01 .REO.0000000000000076

Davies, C., Nitz, A. J., Mattacola, C. G., Kitzman, P., Howell, D., Viele, K., . . . , Brockopp, D. (2014). Practice patterns when treating patients with low back pain: A survey of physical therapists. *Physiotherapy Theory and Practice, 30*(6), 399–408. doi:10.3109/09593985.2013.877547

Davies, C. C., Brockopp, D., & Moe, K. (2016). Astym therapy improves function and range of motion following mastectomy. *Breast Cancer, 8*, 39–45. doi:10.2147/bctt.s102598

Davies, C. C., Brockopp, D., Moe, K., Wheeler, P., Abner, J., & Lengerich, A. (2017). Exploring the lived experience of women immediately following mastectomy: A phenomenological study. *Cancer Nursing, 40*(5), 361–368. doi:10.1097/ncc.0000000000000413

Davies, C. C., & Brockopp, D. Y. (2010). Use of ASTYM® treatment on scar tissue following surgical treatment for breast cancer: A pilot study. *Rehabilitation Oncology, 28*(3), 3–12.

Davies, C. C., Colon, G., Geyer, H., Pfalzer, L., & Fisher, M. I. (2016). Oncology EDGE task force on prostate cancer outcomes: A systematic review of outcome measures for functional mobility. *Rehabilitation Oncology, 34*(3), 82–96. doi:10.1097/01.REO.0000000000000029

Dillman, D., Smyth, J. D., & Christian, L. M. (2009). *Internet, mail and mixed-mode surveys: The tailored design method.* Hoboken, NJ: John Wiley & Sons Inc.

Gilbert, P., Rutland, M. D., & Brockopp, D. (2013). Redesigning the work of case management: Testing a predictive model for readmission. *American Journal of Management Care, 19*(10 Spec No), eS19–eSP25.

Honaker, J., Brockopp, D., & Moe, K. (2014a). Development and psychometric testing of the Honaker suspected deep tissue injury severity scale. *Journal of Wound, Ostomy, and Continence Nursing, 41*(3), 238–241. doi:10.1097/won.0000000000000024

Honaker, J., Brockopp, D., & Moe, K. (2014b). Suspected deep tissue injury profile: A pilot study. *Advanced Skin and Wound Care, 27*(3), 133–140; quiz 141–132. doi:10.1097/01.asw.0000443267.25288.87

Honaker, J., & Forston, M. (2011). Adjunctive use of noncontact low-frequency ultrasound for treatment of suspected deep tissue injury: A case series. *Journal of Wound, Ostomy, and Continence Nursing, 38*(4), 394–403. doi:10.1097/WON.0b013e31821e87eb

Honaker, J. S., Forston, M. R., Davis, E. A., Weisner, M. M., Morgan, J. A., & Sacca, E. (2016). The effect of adjunctive noncontact low frequency ultrasound on deep tissue pressure injury. *Wound Repair and Regeneration, 24*(6), 1081–1088. doi:10.1111/wrr.12479

Honaker, J. S., Forston, M. R., Davis, E. A., Wiesner, M. M., & Morgan, J. A. (2013). Effects of non-contact low-frequency ultrasound on healing of suspected deep tissue injury: A retrospective analysis. *International Wound Journal, 10*(1), 65–72. doi:10.1111/j.1742-481X.2012.00944.x

Kjelland, K., Corley, D., Slusher, I., Moe, K., & Brockopp, D. (2014). The Best for Baby Card: An evaluation of factors that influence women's decisions to breastfeed. *Newborn & Infant Nursing Reviews, 14*(1), 23–27. doi:10.1053/j.nainr.2013.12.007

Lengerich, A., Bugajski, A., Marchese, M., Hall, B., Yackzan, S., Davies, C., & Brockopp, D. (2017). The Baptist Health Nurse Retention questionnaire: A methodological study, part 1. *Journal of Nursing Administration, 47*(5), 289–293. doi:10.1097/nna.0000000000000480

Levenhagen, K., Davies, C., Perdomo, M., Ryans, K., & Gilchrist, L. (2017a). Diagnosis of upper-quadrant lymphedema secondary to cancer: Clinical practice guideline from the oncology section of APTA. *Rehabilitation Oncology, 35*(3), e1–e18. doi:10.1097/01.reo.0000000000000073

Levenhagen, K., Davies, C., Perdomo, M., Ryans, K., & Gilchrist, L. (2017b). Diagnosis of upper quadrant lymphedema secondary to cancer: Clinical practice guideline from the oncology section of the American Physical Therapy Association. *Physical Therapy, 97*(7), 729–745. doi:10.1093/ptj/pzx050

Lewis, C. P., Corley, D. J., Lake, N., Brockopp, D., & Moe, K. (2015). Overcoming barriers to effective pain management: The use of professionally directed small group discussions. *Pain Management Nursing, 16*(2), 121–127. doi:10.1016/j.pmn.2014.05.002

Lewis, D. A., Sanders, L. P., & Brockopp, D. Y. (2011). The effect of three nursing interventions on thermoregulation in low birth weight infants. *Neonatal Networks, 30*(3), 160–164. doi:10.1891/0730-0832.30.3.160

Melton, L., Lengerich, A., Collins, M., McKechan, R., Dunn, D., Griggs, P., . . . , Bugajski, A. (2017). Evaluation of huddles: A multisite study. *Health Care Management, 36*(3), 282–287. doi:10.1097/hcm.0000000000000171

Moe, K., Brockopp, D., McCowan, D., Merritt, S., & Hall, B. (2015). Major predictors of inpatient falls: A multisite study. *Journal of Nursing Administration, 45*(10), 498–502. doi:10.1097/nna.0000000000000241

Polit, D. F., & Beck, C. T. (2017). *Nursing research: Generating and assessing evidence for nursing practice.* Philadelphia, PA: Wolters Kluwer.

Roser, L. P., Piercy, E. C., & Altpeter, T. (2014). Targeting zero: One hospital's journey to reduce CAUTI. *Nursing Management, 45*(12), 18–20. doi:10.1097/01.NUMA.0000456652.02404.b5

Ross, K., Mathis, S., & Brockopp, D. (2008). Developing a successful palliative care service in an acute care setting. *Journal of Nursing Administration, 38*(6), 282–286. doi:10.1097/01.NNA.0000312787.88093.ca

Schreiber, J. A., & Brockopp, D. Y. (2012). Twenty-five years later—what do we know about religion/spirituality and psychological well-being among breast cancer survivors? A systematic review. *Journal of Cancer Survivorship, 6*(1), 82–94. doi:10.1007/s11764-011-0193-7

Schreiber, J. A., Cantrell, D., Moe, K. A., Hench, J., McKinney, E., Preston Lewis, C., . . . , Brockopp, D. (2014). Improving knowledge, assessment, and attitudes related to pain management: Evaluation of an intervention. *Pain Management Nursing, 15*(2), 474–481. doi:10.1016/j.pmn.2012.12.006

Stoltz, R., Byrd, R., Hench, A. J., Slone, T., Brockopp, D., & Moe, K. (2014). Does the type of sleep surface influence infant wellbeing in the NICU? *American Journal of Maternal Child Nursing, 39*(6), 363–368. doi:10.1097/nmc.0000000000000078

Thompson, M., Moe, K., & Lewis, C. P. (2014). The effects of music on diminishing anxiety among preoperative patients. *Journal of Radiology Nursing, 33*(4), 199–202. doi:10.1016/j.jradnu.2014.10.005

Watkins, S., Corley, D., Cleeter, D., Moe, K., & Brockopp, D. (2014). Implementing a nurse leader fellowship model. *Nursing Management, 45*(7), 53–55. doi:10.1097/01.NUMA.0000451038.15082.b7

Watson, J. (2012). *HUMAN caring science: A theory of nursing.* Sudbury, MA: Jones and Bartlett Learning.

Weyl, H., Yackzan, S., Ross, K., Henson, A., Moe, K., & Lewis, C. P. (2015). Understanding colorectal screening behaviors and factors associated with screening in a community hospital setting. *Clinical Journal of Oncology Nursing, 19*(1), 89–93. doi:10.1188/15.cjon.89-93

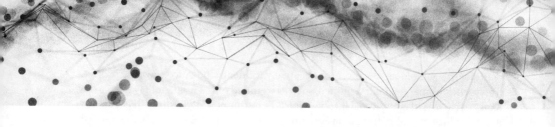

CHAPTER 4

Research Methods in a Research-Friendly Environment: An Overview

"... the world view of science is relational and relativistic and not an absolute separatist view of reality and phenomena."

— **Watson**, 2012

▶ Introduction

This chapter addresses research designs, measurement, sample selection and size, and data collection strategies. Methods are discussed as they relate to studies that involve human subjects. Laboratory research is not addressed. Both quantitative and qualitative approaches to research are presented, and examples of studies conducted in this research-friendly environment (RFE) are included. The Research-Friendly Environment Model (RFEM) presented in Chapter 3 has guided these studies.

The designs associated with both quantitative and qualitative studies provide a foundation for the remainder of the research process. Designs and methods are based on the research question and the desired outcomes of the project. Thoughtful consideration of both can ensure that the problem under examination is adequately and accurately addressed.

This foundation guides the measurement of variables of interest, data collection, construction of an intervention when appropriate, and analysis of data. Effectively measuring the variables of interest is an essential part of the research process—without accurate measurement, data are unlikely to be meaningful. Similarly, the selection and size of a sample can positively or negatively influence the outcome of the project. Interventions may be predetermined, such as a guided ultrasound, or may need to be constructed, as in educational interventions. For example, in the study that assessed the influence of group discussions on nurses' knowledge of pain and biases toward specific patient groups and their pain (Lewis, Corley, Lake, Brockopp, & Moe, 2015), the intervention was carefully structured and described in detail. A goal of carefully constructing interventions is to enable others to replicate a study.

Designs used in both quantitative and qualitative research are described in this chapter. Examples of both types of studies conducted in this RFE are provided. Basic assumptions of both approaches to conducting research are presented. In addition, advantages and disadvantages of experimental designs are included. Four commonly used qualitative designs are described, along with examples of three qualitative studies conducted in this RFE.

Measurement is addressed as it relates to the design of a study and proposed procedures of data collection. Whether to select an instrument from the literature, modify an instrument selected from the literature, or develop a new instrument is discussed. In terms of testing an intervention, guidelines are proposed for selecting or constructing an intervention. Sample size and how to select a sample are also discussed. Chapter 5 addresses measurement in depth, and Chapter 6 describes the application of statistics.

▶ Quantitative Research

For many years, healthcare providers have designated quantitative research methods as the preferred approach to obtaining evidence to support clinical practice. As a result, hospital-based caregivers are likely to favor these methods; caregivers in this RFE lean strongly toward conducting quantitative rather than qualitative research. In addition, educational preparation for caregivers has focused on quantitative approaches to research as the best method for obtaining useful results. In general, the healthcare system has supported a quantitative approach to research (DiCenso, Guyatt, & Ciliska, 2005).

Specifically, the recommendation within healthcare has been to obtain evidence by conducting experimental research, also known as randomized controlled trials (RCTs), whenever possible. To date, RCTs have not been completed in this RFE. There are, however, three RCTs in the data collection phase. While RCTs have been viewed within health care as the gold standard for changing practice, they are neither useful nor feasible in many situations. Given that RCTs may not be feasible in a number of situations, caregivers can still test interventions by using a less stringent design, the quasi-experiment.

The quasi-experiment is a design that caregivers can select when randomization to experimental and control groups is not feasible. Interventions tested and results published in this RFE using quasi-experimental designs include music in a preoperative setting (Thompson, Moe, & Lewis, 2014); occlusive wrap, occlusive wrap plus chemical mattress, and occlusive wrap plus temperature control in a neonatal intensive care unit (NICU; Lewis, Sanders, & Brockopp, 2011); and a laminated, pocket-sized card to encourage breastfeeding in clinical practices associated with the hospital (Kjelland, Corley, Slusher, Moe, & Brockopp, 2014).

While experimental methods (experiments and quasi-experiments) are the preferred approach to research in health care, a descriptive approach can also provide clinically useful information. The aim of descriptive research is to describe or explain phenomena. Findings from descriptive studies can be used to modify practice or lead to the development of interventions that can be tested using an experimental design. When little is known about a patient-care issue, using descriptive methods to better understand the issue can provide a foundation for further investigation. Descriptive studies in this RFE have described factors related to nurse retention (Bugajski et al., 2017), patients' experience of hourly rounding (Bragg et al., 2016), a profile of patients with deep-tissue wound injuries (Honaker, Brockopp, & Moe, 2014), huddles (Melton et al., 2017), and job satisfaction among hospital-based medical imaging technologists (Fultz, Walker, Lengerich, & Bugajski, 2017). Both organizational changes and changes in practice have occurred based on the results of these studies.

Assumptions Underlying Quantitative Research

Quantitative and qualitative approaches to research differ in regard to underlying assumptions. There are three major assumptions that apply to quantitative research: (1) an objective reality exists that can be assessed, (2) the investigator can and should be completely removed from study procedures, and (3) a highly structured process is required in order to gain accurate information. When conducting quantitative research, investigators are required to develop a specific, orderly plan that will guide all research activities. A series of steps is proposed that must be followed in a predetermined order. Bias related to any component of the plan is diminished to the greatest extent possible (Polit & Beck, 2016). Producing empirical evidence (i.e., evidence based in objective reality) is a goal of quantitative research.

To conduct quantitative research, data must be numerical, gathered using a formal measurement process, and analyzed using statistical procedures. The assumptions underlying quantitative research, specifically RCTs, suggest that findings can be generalized to populations other than the sample studied. The generalizability or "external validity" of a study refers to the extent to which the findings of a study can be generalized to a larger population. The ability to generalize findings is a key criterion for evaluating quantitative studies (Polit & Beck, 2016).

Quantitative Research Designs

Experimental and descriptive designs are the two major categories of designs used in quantitative research. The experimental category includes quasi-experiments and RCTs. Exploratory, explanatory, correlational, and case studies are examples of descriptive studies (*descriptive* is used in this text rather than *nonexperimental*).

Caregivers use experimental designs to test interventions. Testing an intervention is often referred to as the "manipulation of a variable." Investigators manipulate one variable, the independent variable, and assess another variable (or variables), the dependent variable. For example, investigators in this RFE have conducted studies examining the effect of music (independent variable) on variables of interest (dependent variables). In one study, Thompson et al. (2014) examined the effect of music (independent variable) on anxiety levels (dependent variable) among patients prior to surgery. Bowles, Curtis, Davies, Bugajski, and Lengerich (2018) also investigated the use of music. They examined the influence of music (independent variable) over a 9-week period on motivation to exercise, differences in distance walked, and mood (dependent variables) among cardiac rehabilitation patients.

Interactions with caregivers in this RFE suggest that intervention studies are frequently their first choice as a research method. Given caregivers' role at the bedside, they become aware, sometimes painfully, of problems with patient care and can often suggest alternative approaches. When they come to the research office with ideas for an alternative approach to care that they would like to evaluate, both RCTs and quasi-experiments are considered. Because randomization to experimental and control groups is not feasible in some situations, and not ethical in others, a quasi-experimental design is often selected.

For example, the two music studies described above were quasi-experiments. Patients in the cardiac rehabilitation study exercised together, side by side. It did not seem desirable in that setting to provide music for some and not for others. Investigators who conducted the study that examined the influence of music on preoperative anxiety needed assistance from staff to supervise the music experience. Patients were in private preoperative bays, and when staff were available, patients who listened to music were placed in the experimental group. Patients who did not have the experience because staff were not available were assigned to the control group. Findings of both studies have resulted in changes in the institution. Music is now offered to all patients.

Experimental Research Designs

RCTs are studies that test the effect of an intervention on specified variables. The intervention or independent variable is examined in relation to one or more dependent variables. The RCT requires participants to be randomly assigned to an experimental group (experiences the intervention) and a control group (does not experience the intervention). Using this design and depending on the degree of control exerted, investigators may infer causality. To date in this RFE, most caregivers working with research consultants have decided that quasi-experiments are better suited to their research questions than RCTs. The funded study discussed in **BOX 4-1**, however, is an ongoing RCT led by a baccalaureate-prepared nurse.

 BOX 4-1 Peggy Wheeler, RN, BSN, OCN: Evaluation of a Post-mastectomy Compression Garment

A representative for the manufacturer of a garment that women wear when horseback riding was approached by a rider who commented on the garment sold by this company. She said she wished the garment had been available to her when she had a mastectomy for breast cancer, commenting that the garment was comfortable and supportive. The representative took the idea to Peggy Wheeler, a nurse navigator in this RFE, to see if a study measuring patient satisfaction with this garment could be conducted. Working with a research consultant, she designed an RCT to evaluate the comfort of this new garment post mastectomy. Peggy and the research consultant negotiated with the manufacturer of the garment to fund the study. Following receipt of informed consent, women are randomized to a control group (wear traditional garment) and an experimental group (wear new garment). Measures related to comfort levels will be collected for a period of time during garment use. By randomly assigning patients to either wear the new garment or the standard one, investigators have the greatest likelihood, in terms of design, of establishing whether or not the new garment improves comfort level. This study is ongoing.

Findings from this study will provide information that can infer causality related to the use of the garment. While a quasi-experiment without randomization could have been conducted, results would not have the same strength in terms of suggesting that the garment was responsible for increased comfort levels. Randomization was ethically appropriate because the present garment provides some degree of comfort, women in the control group do have use of an appropriate garment, and the use of these garments is not detrimental to the women's health. In addition, sufficient staff are available to manage the distribution of garments to each group.

Findings from this study will provide information that can infer causality related to the use of the garment. While a quasi-experiment without randomization could have been conducted, results would not have the same strength in terms of suggesting that the garment was responsible for increased comfort levels.

There are pros and cons related to conducting research using experimental designs. Advantages and disadvantages of both experimental and quasi-experimental designs are presented below.

Advantages. The RCT is considered to be the gold standard in research because optimal control is exerted over all components of the research process. A requirement of this design is to impose sufficient control over variables studied as well as the study environment so that alternative explanations for the outcomes of a study are extremely unlikely. For example, in the study evaluating different compression garments among women following mastectomy, if age of participants is not controlled, results could be related to age differences rather than the garment. In addition to controlling for specific variables such as age, random assignment to control and experimental groups assures as much as possible that participants are similar.

In addition to exerting maximum control over components of the research process, bias related to a particular outcome in quantitative research is not acceptable. Investigators' understanding and acknowledgment of their biases are required when conducting quantitative research. They must consider their biases in relation to their study throughout the data collection process and must do everything possible to diminish bias. In some quantitative studies, in order to diminish possible bias toward an outcome, participants do not know which intervention they are receiving. They are blinded in terms of which drug or protocol they experience so that knowledge of their particular protocol cannot influence outcomes. In addition, sometimes studies are double-blinded, meaning that neither participants nor the investigators know who receives which treatment. In addition to randomizing participants to experimental and control groups, blinding participants and/or investigators diminishes bias further, ensuring that results can be trusted to reflect causation to the greatest degree possible.

The example in **BOX 4-2** is a double-blinded RCT under institutional review board (IRB) review that will compare an ultrasound IPack block with surgeon infiltration of the posterior knee capsule on postoperative pain, opioid and antiemetic consumption, mobility, and length of stay following total knee arthroplasty.

Investigators who conduct RCTs in the healthcare arena tend to focus on the impact of specific treatments, such as the effect of a new drug on an illness or the outcome of a specific treatment protocol. As mentioned previously, the strength of the RCT, when compared to other designs, is the extent of control it affords the researcher over the study environment as well as variables of interest. When conducting an RCT, the following factors must be present: (1) the cause must precede the effect, (2) the

BOX 4-2 John Edwards, RN, CRNA: Effect of an Ultrasound IPack Block on Pain, Opioid and Antimetic, Mobility, and Length of Stay

John and a team of investigators have designed a study to compare an ultrasound IPack block with surgeon infiltration of the posterior knee capsule on patients having total knee arthroplasty. They hypothesize that the block will diminish postoperative pain and opioid and antiemetic use, increase mobility following surgery, and decrease length of stay in the hospital. Patients will be randomly assigned to an experimental group (IPack block) and a control group (standard care—surgeon infiltration of posterior knee capsule). Neither patients nor caregivers will know which patient is receiving which intervention (double-blinded).

effect must be based on the presumed cause, and (3) the effect cannot be due to the influence of a variable other than the one under consideration.

Hypotheses regarding the outcome of both RCTs and quasi-experiments are specified. Usually, the hypothesis states that a difference in a particular direction will occur. For example, investigators in this RFE hypothesized that use of Astym (an approach to working with soft-tissue injuries) would improve upper extremity functioning among women post mastectomy (Davies, Brockopp, & Moe, 2016). Results of the study showed improvements in both range of motion in the involved quadrant and overall functioning in the upper extremity.

Disadvantages. For ethical as well as practical reasons, the degree of control required by an RCT may not be feasible. For example, withholding a known treatment from patients by randomizing participants to a control group in order to test a new, unproven approach to care would not be ethical. In some instances, however, standard treatment can be compared with a new approach; for example, members of the control group in the study described in Box 4-2 will receive standard treatment. Even so, there are situations that do not lend themselves to an RCT. Once there is evidence to suggest that an intervention is useful, it is not ethical to withhold that intervention from participants. In addition, in a hospital setting, randomly assigning patients who share a room to different groups may cause contamination of results.

A requirement of an RCT is to ensure, as much as possible, that individuals in the experimental and control groups are as similar as possible. However, creating artificial circumstances in order to conduct a study can be a disadvantage. Given that most researchers in health care want to make changes in real-life situations, creating a context that is not real may produce inaccurate outcomes.

When artificial requirements are imposed on the design of a study, application of findings becomes questionable. For example, when studying a new protocol for depression, if participation must be limited to individuals diagnosed with a major depressive disorder and no other mental health diagnosis, investigators are creating a situation that does not reflect the real world given that, in practice, it is uncommon for individuals to present only with a major depressive disorder. Because of the artificial circumstances the experiment created, the results of the study may not be of any benefit to clinicians working in the field.

In addition to issues related to the control required by an RCT, resources necessary to complete an RCT may pose a problem. Management of these studies may require staff or investigator time beyond that which is available. Because potential participants may not want to be randomized to a group that does not receive the intervention, enrolling participants may take longer than planned. Also, ensuring that participants in each group remain independent of one another can require additional time and energy. The result is an extra burden on staff and/or increased costs.

Given that results of an RCT are dependent on strict control of both the variables and environment of the study, any intervening uncontrolled event can alter results. A problem called the Hawthorne effect, in which study participants alter their behavior because they know they are participating in a study, can occur in either an RCT or a quasi-experiment. For example, nurses in a study may adhere more carefully to an intervention because they are aware outcomes are being measured.

Quasi-Experimental Research Designs

Similar to RCTs, quasi-experiments are designed to evaluate interventions. Random assignment to experimental and control groups, however, is not required. Quasi-experiments are the most common study design used by researchers in this RFE, because these designs are often more feasible than RCTs and can still imply causation. Depending on the question asked, there are a number of approaches to conducting quasi-experiments. The following section describes advantages and disadvantages of this design.

Advantages. When RCTs are not feasible, investigators who want to test a particular intervention frequently design quasi-experiments. These designs range from simple to complex. A research question may address the effect of one intervention on one variable among one group of participants, or more than one intervention may be involved. In addition, a number of variables may be assessed and the intervention tested within several groups.

Quasi-experiments may be conducted with one group of participants by measuring the dependent variable before and after the intervention (no control group/random assignment). They may also be conducted with two or more groups; however, participants are not randomly assigned to each group.

Conducting a quasi-experiment can enable investigators to resolve ethical and/or practical issues associated with RCTs. The design of a NICU sleep surface study is presented in **BOX 4-3** with reasons for designing a quasi-experiment rather than an RCT.

 BOX 4-3 Regina Stoltz, RN, MSN, APRN: Effect of Two Sleep Surfaces on Nurses' Perception of Infant Sleep Pain, Comfort, Weight, and Vital Signs

In order to evaluate differences in the effect of two sleep surfaces on nurses' perceptions of infant sleep, pain, comfort, weight, and vital signs, Regina designed a quasi-experiment. Following parental consent, data were collected on variables of interest on 40 infants on mattresses in use at the hospital. At the conclusion of data collection, the mattress of interest was available on the unit, and parents could enroll their infants in the study on this second surface. While a control group was a component of the study, randomization did not occur. Parents of these vulnerable infants did not need to consider their baby being randomized to an unknown situation, the unit did not need to put both mattresses in place, and staff were not required to keep track of infant placement in the control or experimental group.

Disadvantages. The internal validity of a study is the extent to which results accurately reflect cause and effect. The internal validity of an experiment is greater than that of a quasi-experiment. The major disadvantage of the quasi-experiment is the lack of control that can be exerted when compared with an RCT. In addition to the lack of randomization, when events beyond the control of the investigator occur simultaneously with the intervention, the internal validity of both designs can be influenced.

For example, nurses played an important role in Regina's quasi-experiment testing the effect of sleep surfaces on infants' well-being (Box 4-3). If a large group of nurses left the hospital during the study, outcomes related to the sleep surfaces would be questionable. In addition, occurrences over time during the study can limit internal validity. A question regarding the sleep surface study is related to the fact that while the study was ongoing, the infants were maturing. The question arises: Could the process of maturation have influenced results?

Experimental and Quasi-Experimental Research Designs: Summary. Quantitative designs are the traditional approach to gaining information that will improve health care. Objectivity, structure, and generalizability are key concepts of this methodology. It is important to note that investigators using these methods do not "prove" a given outcome but simply provide information as to the likelihood that a given outcome is repeatable. Likelihood, or probability, is addressed in detail in Chapter 6.

Descriptive Research Designs

Descriptive designs are not used to test interventions. Investigators conducting these studies may want to understand a particular variable, determine differences between two or more variables, or compare data related to two or more variables. For example, nurse educators might study the knowledge level of a certain aspect of care among bedside caregivers. Another study might examine the relationship between socioeconomic status and well-being among women diagnosed with breast cancer.

Because descriptive studies do not involve the development and application of an intervention, they are generally easier to conduct and require fewer resources. These studies often provide information that leads to the development of interventions. They can also lead to change. For example, Honaker and colleagues' (2014) study on developing a profile of patients with deep-tissue injuries led to the examination of ultrasound as a method for treating these wounds (Honaker et al., 2016). Results led to practice changes within the institution.

Descriptive studies examine existing phenomena and may involve one or more groups of participants. The goal of descriptive quantitative studies is to accurately describe characteristics of a group of individuals or specific situations. Frequencies, relationships, and/or differences of the characteristics studied are presented. Topics of interest to healthcare professionals include health status of specific groups, health-related behaviors, and attitudes toward health and illness. Descriptive studies frequently provide explanations or relationships that permit the development of interventions.

Four types of descriptive studies—exploratory, explanatory, correlational, and case studies—are described in the following pages. Topics examined using descriptive methods in this RFE include nurse retention (Bugajski et al., 2017), well-being of women diagnosed with breast cancer (Davies et al., 2017), hourly rounding (Bragg et al., 2016), huddles (Melton et al., 2017), wound care (Honaker, Brockopp, & Moe, 2014), and colorectal screening (Weyl et al., 2015).

Exploratory Research Designs. Caregivers in this RFE have addressed a variety of issues using descriptive research methods. When little information is available on a particular topic, such as when a new or innovative area of interest is identified, an exploratory design is appropriate. The purpose of an exploratory study may be to provide a foundation for developing an intervention or designing a needed assessment. The goal of investigators who use this approach is to provide a clear description of a particular situation.

Gaining information from descriptive studies is often a useful strategy prior to considering changes in clinical practice. An example of designing a descriptive study in order to intervene regarding a clinical problem is the initial work involved in the development of the Baptist Health High Risk Falls Assessment (BHHRFA). When the incidence of falls increased on a large medical-surgical unit, the unit manager came to a research consultant to discuss how caregivers could be more successful in predicting patients at risk for falling. They reviewed the literature and found that high-risk falls assessments existed, but their ability to predict patient falls was less than desirable. In addition, there was no research that investigated the reasons why patients thought they fell. Before developing another high-risk falls assessment, it seemed appropriate to ask patients why they fell. The study in **BOX 4-4** explored the reasons why falls occurred from the patient's perspective.

Explanatory Research Designs. Investigators use an explanatory design to develop systematic explanations for relationships among variables. Explanatory studies are usually conducted when there is a basic understanding of the topic of interest. Using an explanatory design, investigators can make predictions that may add to a

---

 BOX 4-4 Denise McCowan, RN, MSN: Patients' Perceptions of In-Hospital Falls

In an attempt to reduce the incidence of falls on her unit, Denise met with a research consultant. They discussed the fact that even though a number of fall prevention interventions had been put in place, the incidence of falls was higher than ideal. A review of the literature revealed that investigators of studies on falls reported caregivers' explanations of why patients had fallen, but they had not asked patients why they fell. Denise and the consultant decided that face-to-face interviews with inpatients who fell might provide information not found in outcomes of prior research. Supervisors at four institutions within the same hospital system agreed to use a structured format to interview patients (N=118) immediately after they fell. Factors analyzed from data provided by these interviews, along with factors reported in the literature, were used to develop a high-risk falls assessment. A 5-year multisite study resulted in the development, testing, and publication of the Baptist Health High Risk Falls Assessment (Corley et al., 2014), which is now used in a number of hospitals in the region. In addition, the incidence of falls has diminished. Study findings were also incorporated into unit action plans to increase retention of staff.

body of evidence. For example, nurse retention is an important concern of hospital administrators. Based on evidence, an investigator could predict that practicing in a hospital that provides optimal patient care is an important factor in retaining nurses (Bugajski et al., 2017). That factor could be studied using an explanatory design (see **BOX 4-5**).

Case Studies. The intent of a case study is to explore in detail a real-life situation. One or more cases may be used to provide an in-depth understanding of a particular issue or problem. The case or cases must be described within boundaries such as a particular diagnosis or a specific place or time. The example in **BOX 4-6** describes a case series conducted in this RFE to gain a better understanding of suspected deep-tissue injuries.

Correlational Designs. Correlational designs are neither experimental nor descriptive. Descriptive studies are static, whereas correlational studies involve an examination of relationships among variables. Possible questions addressed using

---

 BOX 4-5 Drew Bugajski, RN, BSN: The Importance of Factors Related to Nurse Retention: Using the Baptist Health Nurse Retention Questionnaire

The purpose of this study was to explain the importance of 12 factors thought to influence nurse retention within this RFE. Nurses (N=279) responded to the Baptist Health Nurse Retention Questionnaire. Data were also collected on generation, degree held, specialty, and nursing experience. Findings revealed that clinical and managerial competence, engagement of managers with their employees, and managerial presence on the unit were key to nurse satisfaction and retention. Contrary to expectations, explanations regarding the demographic data collected showed that generation, degree held, specialty, and nursing experience did not influence nurses' desire to stay in the setting. Although the literature describes Millennials as having a different work ethic and work expectations than others, the variable *generation* did not influence outcomes. Study findings were presented at the annual symposium and published (Bugajski et al., 2017).

 BOX 4-6 Jeremy Honaker, RN, BSN, CWOCN: Adjunctive Use of Noncontact Low-Frequency Ultrasound for Treatment of Suspected Deep-Tissue Injury

Jeremy designed a case series study in order to better understand the role of non-contact low-frequency ultrasound in preventing the progression of suspected deep-tissue injuries (SDTI) to stage 3 or 4 pressure ulcers. Six patients received noncontact low-frequency ultrasound and were studied in detail regarding gender, age, overall health status, present diagnosis, prognosis, treatment, and wound progression. Given the analysis of information related to these six patients, two recommendations were made. The first was to suggest noncontact low-frequency ultrasound as a treatment to halt progression of SDTIs; the second was to recommend that a clinical trial be conducted to provide additional information related to prevention of progression of these wounds. His case series was published in a peer-reviewed journal (Honaker & Forston, 2011). Conducting case studies typically involves accessing multiple sources of information. In the SDTI study, Jeremy used photographs of patients' wounds in addition to other data sources.

correlational designs include the following: What is the relationship between weight and sense of well-being in teenagers? How does job satisfaction relate to nurse retention? What is the relationship between anxiety levels among women in labor and length of contractions?

There are a number of ways to analyze data in terms of relationship. A generally accepted process of data analysis, given questions similar to those above, is to have numerical values associated with each variable. For example, anxiety levels among women in labor could be assessed numerically for each participant, and length of labor could be measured in minutes. These two series of numbers can be analyzed to produce an r value that represents the extent of the relationship between 0 and 1 or 0 and -1.

Descriptive Research Designs: Summary

There are three possible goals of descriptive research: (1) accurate portrayal of specific groups or situations, (2) an explanation of differences among variables, or (3) an explanation of relationships among variables. Studies that examine the relationship between an assessment (e.g., the BHHRFA) and how well it predicts a desired outcome (e.g., inpatient falls) are within the descriptive category of research methods. In addition, examination of the psychometric properties (reliability, validity) is also included in this category.

Several studies to design and test instruments have been conducted in this RFE. Development and psychometric testing of the Honaker Suspected Deep Tissue Injury Severity Scale (Honaker et al., 2014), evaluating preceptors (Bradley et al., 2015), the Baptist Health High Risk Fall Assessment: a methodological study (Corley et al., 2014), and the Baptist Health Nurse Retention Questionnaire: a methodological study (Lengerich et al., 2017) are studies that evaluated relationships between a questionnaire and a desired outcome.

Measurement

Selecting an approach to collecting data and identifying a specific instrument are important steps in designing a study. In relation to collecting data, different approaches may be used depending on the design of the study. Face-to-face or telephone interviews may be used in studies using qualitative or quantitative methods. Paper and pencil questionnaires or questionnaires accessed via computers are generally used in quantitative research. Another approach involves simply counting the number of incidents or activities related to the study purpose. For example, in a study designed to understand colorectal screening behaviors, Weyl et al. (2014) reported the number of individuals who had colorectal screening over a specified period of time.

This chapter describes general principles of measurement in terms of the RFEM. Approximately one-third of research consultants' time in this RFE is spent assisting caregivers to select, modify, or develop an instrument. As health care rapidly changes, the need for instruments to measure new areas related to patient care also increases.

Approaches to Measurement

Face-to-face interviews are often used when the study topic has not been examined and little is known regarding the area of interest. A study examining the influence of massage on neonatal abstinence syndrome (NAS) babies incorporated interviews into the procedure. Mothers of these babies commented on their addiction to drugs, their concern for their infants, and their response to learning about massage.

Many investigators in this RFE use paper and pencil or computer-based questionnaires to gain information related to their topic of interest. There are three possible strategies used to find an instrument to measure a particular area: It may be found in the literature, it may be found in the literature and modified for a purpose that is different from the original intent, or it may be developed to meet a specific need. Purposes for the development of instruments may differ. In this RFE, some instruments have been developed for use across hospital settings, others to answer questions for a specific variable in a specific study, and still others for internal use to address an administrative or clinical question.

While using well-tested instruments is ideal, there is a need to develop and use questionnaires that have not been rigorously tested. At times, particularly when little information related to a variable of interest is available, designing questionnaires without rigorous testing can help investigators gather initial data. For example, Kjelland, Corley, Slusher, Moe, and Brockopp (2014) developed a questionnaire to examine factors related to women's choice to breastfeed. The instrument was designed for a specific use at one point in time.

Five instruments have been designed in this RFE for use across hospital settings. They are an instrument to predict inpatient falls (Corley et al., 2014), an assessment of deep-tissue injuries (Honaker et al., 2014), an instrument to predict dysphagia among pneumonia patients (Groppo-Lawless, Bugajski, Lengerich, & Davies, 2018), an instrument to predict dysphagia post extubation (Moynahan, Swigert, Steele, & Lengerich, 2018), and an evaluation of preceptor performance (Bradley et al., 2015). In addition, four instruments have been developed for use in a specific study. Comfort levels of infants (Stoltz et al., 2014), perceptions of hourly rounding (Bragg et al., 2016), factors related to interest in breastfeeding (Kjelland et al., 2014), and work satisfaction (Fultz et al., 2017) are examples of investigations using this type of instrument.

In relation to internal use, research consultants were asked to design a questionnaire focused on 30-day patient readmissions. The request involved taking an interview designed by a national organization and translating interview questions into structured items that could be responded to by "yes" or "no." The questionnaire was developed for internal use only with no expectation of dissemination of results.

Skills in psychometrics are required to design a questionnaire. There are guidelines for formulating items and rules for developing scales. Investigators need to understand the level of measurement associated with responses to specific items and how data retrieved can be analyzed.

Approaches to Measurement: Summary

Fear of not measuring something the "right way" can keep caregivers from conducting research. When developing an environment that encourages and supports research, it may be important to convey to caregivers that any area of interest can be measured and creative approaches are available. Consultants assist investigators to write items and select appropriate scales. Face-to-face interviews, phone interviews, paper and pencil questionnaires, and electronic surveys are available for caregivers to conduct hospital-based projects.

Sample Size and Selection

An important step in the process of conducting research is determining the population of interest, how the sample will be identified, and how many participants are needed to reach desired outcomes. In a hospital setting, defining a given sample can be difficult. Specific diagnoses may not be grouped on the same unit, and policies regarding visitation and availability may cause problems. Support from administration at all levels is important when designing a study of inpatients. Managers who understand the patient population on a unit where a caregiver is proposing a study can be particularly helpful.

Sample Selection

Participants in studies conducted by hospital-based caregivers can range in age from infancy to the elderly. They may be critically ill or relatively healthy. Study samples in this RFE have included inpatients (Corley et al., 2014), outpatients (Bowles et al., 2018), infants (Stoltz et al., 2014), adult women (Davies et al., 2017), medical imaging technologists (Fultz et al., 2018), and nurses (Bugajski et al., 2017). While caregivers may be clear regarding their population of interest, they may not understand the research requirement for consistency across important participant characteristics. Inclusion and exclusion criteria are addressed prior to accessing a sample.

Inclusion and exclusion criteria are important considerations when deciding how to select a sample. For example, in a study on thermoregulation in low birthweight infants (Lewis et al., 2011), the investigator had to decide what "low birthweight" meant and ensure that only babies at that weight could participate in the study. In all studies in this RFE, participants must speak English and be able to understand the instructions and process. Additional inclusion or exclusion criteria may be developed based on the question asked and the consistency of sample membership required.

If the sample of interest is not randomly selected, decisions must be made as to how selection will occur. The term *convenience sample* is frequently used, implying that a strict regimen has not been used. Some investigators will collect data on all participants over a given period of time. Others will, based on availability, collect data on two specific days per week. Whatever the choice, a plan needs to be developed, and consultants, along with administrators, can assist investigators to access and collect data from the identified sample.

Sample Size

Sample size can vary considerably. In this RFE, sample sizes have varied from 290,000 participants in the study to design and test an inpatient high-risk falls assessment (Corley et al., 2014) to a study that examined an intervention to improve the management of pain involving 32 critical care nurses (Lewis, Corley, Lake, Brockopp, & Moe, 2015). The study that developed the high-risk falls assessment required a large sample size in order to develop an instrument that would have strong predictability,

BOX 4-7 Preston Lewis, RN, DNP, CCRN: Overcoming Barriers to Effective Pain Management: The Use of Professionally Directed Small Group Discussion

Preston wanted to test the effect of professionally led small groups on critical care nurses' knowledge of pain management and their biases toward specific patient populations when managing pain. The hospital unit selected for this project had 12 beds and 34 nurses. All nurses were willing to participate; however, two left the hospital during the study. Preston found that knowledge and biases changed (significantly) in a positive direction following the intervention. His sample plan consisted of focusing on one critical care unit and enrolling all nurses if possible. His results are published (Lewis et al., 2015), and changes in practice based on his study have resulted.

but meaningful information can be obtained using small samples depending on the question addressed. The pain study is described in **BOX 4-7**.

Findings of quantitative studies with small samples selected on the basis of feasibility frequently produce useful results. Changes in nursing care (Kjelland et al., 2014), wound care (Honaker et al., 2014), and nurse preceptor activities (Bradley et al., 2015) have occurred within this setting based on study results. In addition, changes have been made based on these studies at other institutions. For example, Bradley et al. (2015) have received 25 requests from other organizations to use the preceptor evaluation they designed.

In relation to sample size, a formula (power analysis) frequently used in this RFE to identify a sample size is described in Chapter 6. Using this formula, investigators can calculate a sample size that will reflect the likelihood that a significant difference in their results will occur.

Sample Size and Selection: Summary

Selecting the sample of interest and deciding how many participants are needed are important steps when designing a study. In the hospital setting, feasibility is an important consideration. Practical issues, such as how to approach potential participants and what assistance might be required on a unit, need to be assessed. For example, thinking through issues of sample size and selection involved in studying palliative care patients may be different from strategies used to do the same with healthy caregivers.

Quantitative Research: Summary

Caregivers conducting research in a hospital setting have generally adhered to the traditional science approach to investigating questions of interest. This approach emphasizes the importance of objectivity and facts. Numerical in nature, it is concerned with measuring the smallest, most clearly defined parts of a given concept or situation.

Outcomes of quantitative methods are usually viewed as the evidence required in order to change practice. While the use of quantitative methods is important to the advancement of clinical practice, other approaches to collecting and analyzing data can lead to productive change. Investigators may choose to use both quantitative and qualitative methods in a specific study. The ability to generalize results using quantitative methods is a strength of that approach; however, qualitative methods can address concepts in a depth not possible using quantitative methods (Watson, 2012). Of the 45 publications in peer-reviewed journals submitted from this RFE over the past 5 years, 31 are data based. Of these 31 publications, two describe studies that are qualitative in design (Davies et al., 2017; Hahn et al., 2015).

▶ Qualitative Research

Research consultants assist caregivers to decide whether quantitative or qualitative methods would best suit the purpose of their study. These decisions are based on the assumptions underlying the two approaches as well as desired outcomes of the proposed study. Once the decision is made to use a qualitative approach, discussion follows as to what specific qualitative method will be used.

An overview of qualitative methods is presented here. For an in-depth description of the history of qualitative research, its philosophical background, and a comprehensive review of all qualitative designs, readers are referred to other texts (Creswell, 2013; Patton, 2015; Streubert & Carpenter, 2011). Although quantitative methods may be a caregiver's preferred approach to research, the topic under investigation is the driving force in determining whether to use quantitative or qualitative methods.

Assumptions Underlying Qualitative Research

According to Creswell (2013), qualitative research differs fundamentally from quantitative research. Qualitative methods are used to explore a phenomenon in depth, while quantitative methods are used to explain an outcome related to an examination of specific variables. He cites the following four basic assumptions underlying qualitative approaches to research: multiple realities can lead to a meaningful description of a phenomenon, subjective experiences with participants are desirable, biases exist and can be clearly described, and results of qualitative research emerge over time. Another assumption is that findings of qualitative research are not intended to provide information that can be generalized to other settings (Patton, 2015).

The notion of multiple realities can refer to the desirability, when using qualitative methods, of retrieving different responses to the same question. Investigators report differing perspectives regarding the same issue as they develop themes. For example, in Davies and colleagues' (2016) study on women's experience of viewing their mastectomy scars for the first time, one woman was simply glad to be alive, while another was appalled at the sight of her scars. Both responses were viewed as important and informative. Collectively, comments conveyed the great difficulty women had looking at their scars following this surgery.

Bias is thought to be a negative factor when conducting quantitative research. For example, in the anesthesia study described in Box 4-2, neither participants nor caregivers knew which patient was receiving which treatment. These actions are taken in order to diminish bias (Edwards et al., 2018). An assumption of qualitative methods is that investigators are involved but will clearly delineate their "biases" or "value systems" related to the study. Investigators in the breast cancer study (Davies et al., 2016) and the NAS study (Hahn et al., 2016) clarified their values in terms of their clinical experiences with patients prior to conducting their studies. Concern, over time, for women examining their mastectomy for the first time and mothers of NAS infants was experienced by these investigators, but they were aware that they could not permit these concerns to influence the conduct of their studies. Their beliefs that something could be done to alleviate emotional pain associated with both situations led them to conduct their research.

In relation to the importance of subjective evidence, when conducting qualitative research, the closer the participant is to the phenomenon under investigation, the better the outcome. Hahn et al. (2016), in their study of mothers of NAS babies, worked with women in the hospital immediately following the birth of their infants. They taught mothers how to massage their babies and listened to their responses to the activity as well as concerns regarding having an opioid-addicted infant. In both the NAS study and the breast cancer study, participants were interviewed in the setting where they received care and caregivers collected the data. Another difference between quantitative and qualitative research relates to time: while data may be collected over time when using quantitative methods, results are not analyzed until the conclusion of the study. Given qualitative methods, results can emerge during the data collection period.

Quantitative research requires investigators to develop a highly structured plan that is followed without deviation. When using qualitative methods, the question under investigation may change as data are collected. This change in the focus of the study may be due to the fact that little or no information is available on the topic of interest in many qualitative studies, and so even small amounts of new information can lead to large changes. In addition, while a goal of quantitative research is to have as much similarity among specified characteristics as possible, participants in qualitative studies may be purposefully selected to identify a small group of individuals who may differ in a number of characteristics.

To summarize, assumptions underlying qualitative research differ in important ways from the assumptions underlying quantitative research. Immersion and distance are two constructs that differentiate these two approaches to gaining useful information. When conducting quantitative research, distance from participants and objectivity are key assumptions underlying the approach. Qualitative research, however, requires investigators to be immersed in the activity. Bias is viewed by investigators conducting quantitative research as a negative, while investigators conducting qualitative research view bias as ever present and requiring acknowledgment and clarification.

Types of Qualitative Research

As caregivers seek help to design a study in order to answer a question of interest, a discussion of potential methods can be helpful. Available information on the area of interest, the caregiver's knowledge regarding qualitative methods, and the feasibility of conducting a study that may involve considerable time interviewing participants or require frequent visits are topics for conversation. Once the decision has been made to use qualitative methods, an examination of various approaches is warranted. References such as Creswell (2013) and Patton (2015) can be provided for caregivers to gain an understanding of different ways of conducting a study.

Phenomenology, grounded theory, ethnography, and case study are four frequently used approaches to qualitative research. These approaches, although different in some ways, tend to be consistent regarding their differences from quantitative research in terms of the research process. Data are collected in a natural setting, researchers are involved in the study and usually collect data themselves, multiple methods of data collection may be used for the same study, and both inductive and deductive reasoning may be used. Two qualitative studies conducted and published within this RFE are phenomenological in design (Davies et al., 2017; Hahn et al., 2015). The investigator of the third study used a case study approach (Honaker & Forston, 2013).

Phenomenology

While there are a number of schools of thought regarding phenomenological research, describing the "lived experience" or finding the "essence" of a phenomenon are phrases used to characterize this approach. Data are collected on individuals who have experienced a phenomenon to discover "what" they experienced and "how" they experienced it (Creswell, 2015). For example, in the Hahn et al. (2016) study, the goal of the project was to discover what kind of experience was associated with being a mother of a child suffering from opioid withdrawal. The question was, "How did these mothers experience this particular situation?" Similarly, in the Davies et al. (2016) study regarding women's experience following mastectomy, investigators wanted to understand the "essence" or internal response to examining an unattractive mastectomy scar for the first time.

Typically, when conducting phenomenological research, investigators ask broad, general questions. Questions are open-ended, and investigators enable participants to describe their experience. Interviews are usually taped and transcribed. When analyzing data, investigators must be aware of their own biases toward the particular topic and be able to suspend their judgments throughout the analysis process. Transcriptions are read a number of times, usually by two or more individuals. Meaningful phrases and commonality of themes are identified. After a separate analysis by each researcher, the group comes together to reach consensus regarding themes revealed from the data. The process of analysis is time consuming and requires great attention to the detail reported in the transcripts (Polit & Hungler, 2006). Davies et al. (2016) conducted a study using phenomenology to better understand women's response to viewing their mastectomy scars for the first time (**BOX 4-8**).

Grounded Theory

The purpose of a grounded theory approach to research is to develop a theory that explains a social process. For example, a graduate student recently proposed a grounded theory study that would examine how religion in Appalachia influences healthcare

 BOX 4-8 Claire Davies, PT, PhD: Exploring the Lived Experience of Women Immediately Following Mastectomy—a Phenomenological Study

Claire was concerned regarding the number of women who had difficulty looking at their mastectomy scars. Recent research regarding this issue was not available, so she designed a study, using methods derived from phenomenology, to investigate how women responded to this particular situation. She purposely selected a sample of 10 women who would reflect differing ages and marital status. The following eight themes emerged from the data: lasting impact, personal impact, relational impact, gratitude, support system, coping strategies, timing, and discomfort. Findings from this study suggest that women viewing their mastectomy scars for the first time may need additional support. They may also need preparation in terms of what they might experience before looking at their scars (Davies et al., 2017).

practices. Her goal was to develop a theory that would explain activities related to maintaining health as they are influenced by religious beliefs.

Characteristics of grounded theory studies include posing broad questions, reviewing the literature for gaps in information rather than pertinent information related to the phenomenon of interest, an evolving methodology (asking questions, modifying ideas), and a highly structured approach to coding and analyzing data. Following the development of a theory using grounded theory, components of the theory or the theory itself may be tested using quantitative methods in order to assess generalizability (Creswell, 2013). To date, this qualitative method has not been used in this RFE.

Ethnography

Unlike a grounded theory approach, ethnographers begin with a theory of interest. Their goal is to examine the values, beliefs, and/or behaviors of a group of individuals, who belong to a "culture-sharing" group. Ethnographers identify patterns that reflect the group's way of life (Creswell, 2013). For example, a nursing student designed an ethnographic study focused on the infant care practices among members of an indigenous group of women. She found that these women were so committed to child rearing that their pattern of breastfeeding was consistent across the group and considered a requirement of motherhood. This finding does not agree with research conducted in the southeastern United States (Kjelland et al., 2014).

Ethnography does not need to involve indigenous groups of individuals—any group that holds the same values and behaviors can be studied using this method. Hospitals have groups of caregivers that share strong values and patterns of behaviors; groups of those individuals could be studied given an interest in their particular way of functioning. Investigators in this RFE have not yet used ethnography to conduct a study.

Qualitative Research: Summary

Although studies using qualitative methods represent less than 5% of studies designed in this RFE, as qualitative research gains acceptance in health care, that number may increase. Findings of studies using qualitative methods can contribute to improving patient care along with more traditional quantitative approaches. The study on NAS babies and the study on women following mastectomy have led to practice changes and publication. The work on SDTIs continued and resulted in practice changes, plus four additional studies and publications (Honaker & Forston, 2011; Honaker, Forston, Davis, Weisner, & Morgan, 2013; Honaker, Brockopp, & Moe, 2014a; Honaker, Brockopp, & Moe, 2014b; Honaker et al., 2016).

▶ Chapter Summary

A carefully drafted foundation or plan is necessary in order to conduct studies using each of the research methods described in this chapter. Understanding major categories such as quantitative versus qualitative, experimental designs as opposed to quasi-experiments, and phenomenological approaches as opposed to ethnography is important to the success of caregivers' projects.

Consultants and caregivers initiate a project by outlining the research question, identifying methods to be used, and developing a procedure for data collection. At completion of the study, consultants continue to work with investigators to plan for the dissemination of results. Chapter 7 details the process used in this RFE to assist investigators to disseminate their results through publication in peer-reviewed journals.

References

Bowles, L., Curtis, J., Davies, C., Lengerich, A., & Bugajski, A. (2018). Effect of music on mood, motivation and physical exercise in cardiac rehabilitation patients. Manuscript submitted for publication.

Bradley, H., Cantrell, D., Dollahan, K., Hall, B., Lewis, P., Merritt, S., . . . , White, D. (2015). Evaluating preceptors: A methodological study. *Journal for Nurses in Professional Development, 31*(3), 164–169. doi:10.1097/nnd.0000000000000166

Bragg, L. Bugajski, A., Marchese, M., Caldwell, R., Houle, L., Thompson, R., . . . , Lengerich, A. (2016). How do patients perceive hourly rounding? *Nursing Management, 47*(11), 11–13. doi:10.1097/01.NUMA.0000502807.60295.c5

Bugajski, A., Lengerich, A., Marchese, M., Hall, B., Yackzan, S., Davies, C., & Brockopp, D. (2017). The importance of factors related to nurse retention: Using the Baptist Health Nurse Retention questionnaire, part 2. *Journal of Nursing Administration, 47*(6), 308–312. doi:10.1097/nna.0000000000000486

Bugajski, A., Lengerich, A., McCowan, D., Merritt, S., Moe, K., Hall, B., . . . , Brockopp, D. (2017). The Baptist Health High-Risk Falls Assessment: One assessment fits all. *Journal of Nursing Care Quality, 32*(2), 114–119. doi:10.1097/ncq.0000000000000220

Corley, D., Brockopp, D., McCowan, D., Merritt, S., Cobb, T., Johnson, B., . . . , Hall, B. (2014). The Baptist Health High Risk Falls Assessment: A methodological study. *Journal of Nursing Administration, 44*(5), 263–269. doi:10.1097/nna.0000000000000065

Creswell, J. W. (2013). *Qualitative inquiry & research design: Choosing among five approaches.* (3rd ed.). Los Angeles, CA: Sage.

Davies, C., Brockopp, D., & Moe, K. (2016). Astym therapy improves function and range of motion following mastectomy. *Breast Cancer, 8*(1), 39–45. doi:10.2147/bctt.s102598

Davies, C. C., Brockopp, D., Moe, K., Wheeler, P., Abner, J., & Lengerich, A. (2017). Exploring the lived experience of women immediately following mastectomy: A phenomenological study. *Cancer Nursing, 40*(5), 361–368. doi:10.1097/ncc.0000000000000413

Dicenso, A., Guyatt, G., & Ciliska, D. (2005). *Evidence-based nursing: A guide to clinical practice.* St. Louis, MO: Elsevier, Mosby.

Fultz, A, Walker, M., Lengerich, A., & Bugajski, A. (2018). Job satisfaction of medical imaging technologists: A current look at work environment, communication and leadership. Manuscript submitted for publication.

Groppo-Lawless, S., Bugajski, D., & Davies C. (2018). Development of the Baptist Health dysphagia screen for patients diagnosed with pneumonia. Manuscript submitted for publication.

Hahn, J., Byrd, R., Lengerich, A., Hench, J., Ford, C., Byrd, S., & Stoltz, R. (2015). Neonatal abstinence syndrome: The experience of infant massage. *Creative Nursing, 22*(1), 45–50. doi:10.1891/1078-4535.22.1.45

Honaker, J., & Forston, M. (2011). Adjunctive use of noncontact low-frequency ultrasound for treatment of suspected deep tissue injury: A case series. *Journal of Wound, Ostomy, and Continence Nursing, 38*(4), 394–403. doi:10.1097/WON.ObO13e31821e87eb

Honaker, J. S., Forston, M. R., Davis, E. A., Wiesner, M. M., & Morgan, J. A. (2013). Effects of non-contact low-frequency ultrasound on healing of suspected deep tissue injury: A retrospective analysis. *International Wound Journal, 10*(1), 65–72. doi:10.1111/j.1742-481X.2012.00944.x

Honaker, J., Brockopp, D., & Moe, K. (2014). Development and psychometric testing of the Honaker suspected deep tissue injury severity scale. *Journal of Wound, Ostomy, and Continence Nursing, 4*(12), 238–241. doi:10.1891/0730-0832.30.3.160

Kjelland, K., Corley, D., Slusher, I., Moe, K., & Brockopp, D. (2014). The best for baby card: An evaluation of factors that influence women's decisions to breastfeed. *Newborn & Infant Nursing Reviews, 14*(1), 23–27. doi:10.1053/j.nainr.2013.12.007

Lewis, C. P., Corley, D. J., Lake, N., Brockopp, D., & Moe, K. (2015). Overcoming barriers to effective pain management: The use of professionally directed small group discussions. *Pain Management Nursing, 16*(2), 121–127. doi:10.1016/j.pmn.2014.05.002

Lewis, D. A., Sanders, L. P., & Brockopp, D. Y. (2011). The effect of three nursing interventions on thermoregulation in low birth weight infants. *Neonatal Network, 30*(3), 160–164.

Lengerich, A., Bugajski, A., Marchese, M., Hall, B., Yackzan, S., Davies, C., & Brockopp, D. (2017). The Baptist Health Nurse Retention questionnaire: A methodological study, part 1. *Journal of Nursing Administration, 47*(5), 289–293. doi:10.1097/NNA.0000000000000480

Melton, L., Lengerich, A., Collins, M., McKeehan, R., Dunn, D., Griggs, P., . . . , Bugajski, A. (2017). Evaluation of huddles: A multisite study. *Health Care Management, 36*(3), 282–287. doi:10.1097/hcm.0000000000000171

Patton, M. Q. (2015). *Qualitative research and evaluation methods.* Thousand Oaks, CA: Sage.

Polit, D. F., & Beck C. T. (2017). Nursing research: Generating and assessing evidence for nursing practice. Philadelphia, PA: Wolters Kluwer.

Stoltz, R., Byrd, R., Hench, A. J., Slone, T., Brockopp, D., & Moe, K. (2014). Does the type of sleep surface influence infant wellbeing in the NICU? *American Journal of Maternal Child Nursing, 39*(6), 363–368. doi:10.1097/nmc.0000000000000078

Thompson, M., Moe, K., & Lewis, C. P. (2014). The effects of music on diminishing anxiety among preoperative patients. *Journal of Radiology Nursing, 33*(4), 199–202. doi:10.1016/j.jradnu.2014.10.005

Watson, J. (2012). *Human caring science: A theory of nursing.* Sudbury, MA: Jones and Bartlett Learning.

Weyl, H., Yackzan, S., Ross, K., Henson, A., Moe, K., & Lewis, C. P. (2015). Understanding colorectal screening behaviors and factors associated with screening in a community hospital setting. *Clinical Journal of Oncology Nursing, 19*(1), 89–93. doi:10.1188/15.cjon.89-93.

CHAPTER 5

Measurement: A Model for Instrument Development

"To effectively carry out evidence-based practice, sufficient exploration, research, and evidence gathering must have been generated with regard to the specific clinical issue or case."

— **Porter-O'Grady**, 2010

▶ Introduction

Measurement plays an essential role in nursing and allied health research. This is particularly true as research findings are increasingly expected to impact practice. As a result, understanding how a construct is measured is important. In quantitative research, a construct or specific attribute is referred to as a variable. According to Polit and Beck (2016), a variable is "an attribute that varies, that is, takes on different values." (p. 58). Variables can be objective in nature, such as heart rate and age, or subjective, such as anxiety and well-being.

This chapter describes basic measurement principles that can assist caregivers to select, modify, or develop a measure to assess a variable of interest. The process of selection is, in part, based on a comprehensive literature review. Modification and/ or development of an instrument requires a basic knowledge of psychometrics, the theory underlying principles of measurement. In this chapter, basic principles are conveyed using examples of studies conducted in this research-friendly environment (RFE). The purpose for measuring a variable is discussed, and differences in the rigor of testing instruments are addressed.

In quantitative research, the variables of interest are number-based, meaning that each variable is quantifiable and based on a set of rules. There are two basic rules/ concepts that an investigator must consider when developing an instrument: repeatability (reliability) and accuracy (validity; Nunnally, 1975). These rules constitute the basis for assessing the quality of an instrument. They also serve as guidelines when constructing an instrument.

Self-report measures are frequently used in nursing and allied health research. The two major categories of self-report measures are norm referenced and criterion referenced (Waltz, Strickland, & Lenz, 2010). Norm referenced refers to a comparison between an individual performance and another individual with an "expected" normal performance. Comparing the performance of one individual to a hypothetically average individual is the desired outcome of norm-referenced instruments. For example, a study performed in this RFE that examined the psychological well-being of women with breast cancer, which compared study participants to a sample of nondiagnosed women with similar age/demographics, would be norm referenced (Lengerich et al., 2018). Conversely, criterion-referenced measures provide information that permits a comparison of individuals' responses to a set of predetermined criteria. An instrument that assesses the severity of deep tissue injuries is an example of a criterion-referenced measure. The criteria for grading deep tissue injuries are standard (Honaker, Brockopp, & Moe, 2014).

Anecdotal data collected at this institution, over a 10-year period, suggest that caregivers can have a number of misconceptions regarding measurement. Although dismissing existing instruments as not appropriate is cited as a common error related to measurement (Streiner & Norman, 2008), that is not the experience in this RFE. For example, when an instrument that clearly reflects a given area of interest is not available in the literature, caregivers will often suggest using one that is related, rather than modifying the available instrument or developing a new questionnaire. Their rationale is that they were taught to use published, well-tested measures. Developing their own instrument is viewed as much too difficult and therefore not an option.

Another misconception is related to the use of subscales and the calculation of total scores. In this RFE, several caregivers have not understood the importance of developing categories of items (subscales) and/or developing instruments that permit the calculation of a total score. Caregivers at times develop questionnaires with 20 to 30 items and want to analyze responses to each item. They are not aware that principles of measurement guide investigators to focus on a particular variable. An important component of the measurement process is to focus clearly and specifically on that variable.

Rarely does analyzing a large number of items individually provide useful information. For example, caregivers could design a 30-item instrument to measure nurse satisfaction. Within those 30 items, 10 questions may focus on the work environment as it relates to nurse satisfaction, 10 items may be related to leadership, and the remaining questions may address work–life balance. Information gained from a subset of questions (e.g., leadership) may be more useful and easily reportable than all of the responses as a whole. In addition, if a total score is available, that score can be used to synthesize information and provide a number that can be used to compare with other variables.

Given the number of baccalaureate-prepared caregivers in this RFE who are actively involved in research, these misconceptions may be due to a lack of formal preparation in psychometrics. It has not, however, been difficult for research consultants to teach new researchers, at all levels of educational preparation, how to modify an existing instrument or develop a new one. Following the steps in the Hospital-Based Measurement Model, caregivers have been successful in learning how to effectively measure their variables of interest.

▶ Measurement: A Model for Instrument Development

The Hospital-Based Measurement Model (HBMM) (**FIGURE 5-1**) is the guide used in this RFE when selecting, modifying, or developing an instrument. This model has enabled consultants to assist caregivers to learn how to measure their particular variable

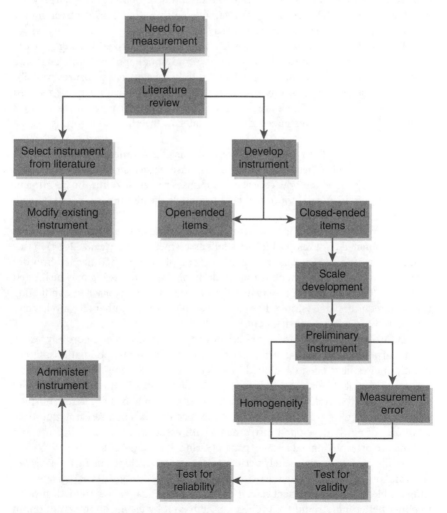

FIGURE 5-1 The Hospital-Based Measurement Model.

of interest. While basic principles are presented in this text, readers are referred to measurement textbooks for details on statistical analyses related to developing an instrument and greater detail regarding the measurement process (Norman & Streiner, 2009; Waltz, Strickland, & Lenz, 2010).

Need for Measurement

Need for
measurement

Given continuous and rapid changes in health care, there is an ongoing need to measure a number of new areas of interest. For example, given that women are now living longer following a mastectomy, the concern for the sequelae of this operation is increasing. Appearance of scar tissue and discomfort following this surgery are variables of interest (Davies, 2017). For variables such as these, prior research may not have been conducted, and measures may not be available.

The need to base care on data is increasingly emphasized throughout the healthcare system. Scientific observation, the traditional approach to examining healthcare problems, requires objectivity. Carefully constructed measures contribute to that requirement. Objectivity of information suggests that instruments need to be rigorously tested. There are, however, degrees of rigor when testing a new questionnaire. In some instances, discussed later in the chapter, rigorous testing is not conducted.

Reliability and validity are the key components of instrument development and evaluation. Reliability reflects to what degree responses to an instrument are repeatable over time. It also refers to how consistent responses to items within the instrument are similar. Validity is a description of how accurately the instrument measures what it was designed to measure.

Rigor refers to how well an instrument has been tested. For example, a 5-year project conducted to develop a high-risk falls assessment (Corley et al., 2014) in this RFE is an example of rigorous testing. A large sample size is often needed in order to rigorously test an instrument. Although desirable, rigorous testing may be limited by the number of available participants. Cost may also be a factor when conducting tests that require a large sample. The purpose of the study is another factor related to the rigor of testing a new instrument.

In this RFE, questionnaires have been developed that have been rigorously tested. Their purpose has been to develop assessments for use across populations. Other questionnaires have been developed in order to conduct a one-time examination of a specific variable for a specific study. Six studies in this RFE were designed and rigorously tested in order to develop instruments that could be used across hospital settings, and five were developed to meet the specific goals of a research question. Examples of newly developed instruments with associated tests of reliability and validity are presented in Tables 5-1 (page 119) and 5-2 (page 120).

While measurement is rarely perfect, instruments developed using a clear set of rules and procedures can provide reasonably precise information. As caregivers confront problems related to patient care, they may want to engage in a systematic process to either better understand the problem or address it by testing an intervention. In response to concerns regarding patient care, they may want to describe health- related phenomena, examine organizational problems, or test an existing instrument.

Once a research question is clearly specified, measures need to be identified within the literature and used as published or modified to fit a specific purpose, or new measures need to be developed. Within this RFE, 10 studies involving investigator-designed instruments have been conducted. The purpose of six studies was to develop a specific instrument for use across acute care institutions (Bradley et al., 2015; Corley et al., 2014; Groppo-Lawless, Davies, Lengerich, & Bugajski, 2018; Honaker, Brockopp, & Moe, 2014; Lengerich et al., 2017; Moynahan, 2018). Four studies addressed attributes that had not been previously measured; investigators in these studies developed questionnaires to assess their specific interest areas (Bragg et al., 2016; Fultz, Walker, Lengerich, & Bugajski, 2017; Kjelland, Corley, Slusher, Moe, & Brockopp, 2014; Stoltz et al., 2018).

The HBMM guides the development of instruments in this RFE. Differences in the time and effort devoted to developing each instrument depend on the goal of the study and vary considerably. For example, developing a tool to predict patients at high risk for falling took 5 years (Corley et al., 2014). The study was conducted in two phases, and both validity (accuracy) and reliability (repeatability, internal consistency) were evaluated. In a different study, the aim was to conduct an initial evaluation of job satisfaction among medical imaging technologists. For this, a questionnaire was completed in several weeks (Fultz & Walker, 2017).

Need for Measurement: Summary

Helping caregivers to specify their purpose in examining a particular construct is an important component of the measurement process. Research consultants can assist caregivers to define and focus on the particular variable(s) they want to measure. Consultants can also assist them to identify available measures, modify a measure if appropriate, or develop a new measure. Consultants often meet with reluctance among caregivers to construct a new instrument, as caregivers have been taught that it is a lengthy, very involved, and difficult process. Consultants work hard to dispel that notion.

Literature Review

Literature
review

A literature review is generally a requirement for decision making related to measurement. Unless a caregiver has selected a specific instrument that will adequately measure the variables under examination, a comprehensive literature review is the first step in the process. Topics of interest can vary greatly. For example, in this RFE, literature reviews in relation to how investigators will assess their clinical constructs of interest have been conducted on deep tissue injuries (Honaker, 2014), factors influencing breastfeeding (Kjelland et al., 2014), and pain management (Schreiber et al., 2014). Organizational issues include the use of huddles in a hospital setting (Melton, 2017) and factors influencing nurse retention (Lengerich et al., 2018).

In each case, the purpose of the literature search was to better understand the construct of interest and to find any existing measures that assess that construct. Objectively measuring a particular variable is the goal of studies using quantitative methods. When variables have not been previously measured or there is little consistency across measures, objectively measuring a variable of interest can be a challenge. An investigator must establish or develop a conceptual definition of their variable of interest, which is an important component of the measurement process. Conceptual definitions are the theoretical or abstract foundation for the meaning given to specific variables.

Examples measured in this RFE include comfort, well-being, and satisfaction. Investigators need to translate these and other concepts of interest into concrete, observable constructs (Waltz, Strickland, & Lenz, 2010). There are many definitions of comfort as this term applies to patients and little agreement as to how it can be assessed. (In contrast, variables such as "falls" can be readily defined; a patient fall is defined at the federal level as an unplanned descent to the floor with or without injury to the patient [Agency for Healthcare Research and Quality, 2013]). In one study, comfort was defined as parents' response to their baby's behaviors (Stoltz et al., 2014). In this study, conducted in this RFE, the effect of sleep surface was examined in relation to infant's well-being (Stoltz et al., 2014). Comfort was defined and measured as follows. My baby seemed irritable/restless was scored as 1, somewhat comfortable 2, and very comfortable 3.

Caregivers frequently want to assess the extent of a given concept in a particular population. They may have a global concept in mind without thinking about the complexity of their area of interest. For example, measuring patient satisfaction can involve physical concerns, psychological issues, and/or social experiences. It is important for the caregiver to determine if he or she wants to examine one or all three areas. Time spent addressing specific meanings of each area through a comprehensive literature review can be helpful.

An example of beginning with a concept—here, psychological well-being—and the process of defining that concept and searching for a measure is presented in **BOX 5-1**. There are several definitions of the construct "psychological well-being." This construct may be defined in terms of the absence of depression or negative feelings or

 BOX 5-1 Alex Lengerich, MS, EdS: Women's Psychological Well-Being Pre- and Post-Diagnosis of Breast Cancer: A Prospective Cohort Study

As a group of investigators gathered to design a study regarding the well-being of women pre- and post diagnosis of breast cancer, they discussed the attribute of interest: "psychological well-being." A search of the literature had revealed a number of definitions and associated measures of this construct. Prior research, to a great extent, had focused on well-being as a lack of distress. Ryff and Singer (1998), however, had developed a definition of well-being from a positive functioning perspective. Their definition was based on the presence of positive affect as opposed to a lack of negative affect. Investigators decided to use that definition for their study. They also used Ryff's questionnaire to assess well-being (Lengerich et al., submitted for publication).

as a positive view of life. The conceptual definition forms the basis for determining what will be measured, and the operational definition refers to the variable in terms of how it will be measured.

Select Instrument from the Literature

Select instrument
from literature

When instruments measuring the topic of interest are available in the literature, it is recommended that investigators contact the author and obtain permission to use the instrument. Investigators who have developed and published instruments may want to charge for its use, some may want access to data collected in order to support or modify their work, and others may give permission to use their instrument without limitations. For example, the nurse who led the project to develop a preceptor evaluation in this RFE (Bradley et al., 2014) has received 25 requests to use her instrument. Two of those requests came from individuals who wanted to modify the instrument. These individuals did not understand that the testing of this instrument would no longer be applicable if the instrument was modified. The author has responded affirmatively to all requests and has informed individuals who want to use the instrument that modifying items has a downside: If modified, the instrument would need to be retested for reliability and validity.

Instruments to measure a construct that an investigator wants to examine may not exist or are considered inadequate for a given purpose. While a search for a tested instrument that will measure the variable of interest is the first step in the measurement process, modifying an available instrument or developing a new one is also an option. Approximately one-third of a research consultant's time in this RFE is spent working with caregivers to assist them in modifying or developing instruments.

Two important criteria for evaluating instruments, validity and reliability, are not characteristics of the instrument itself but reflect how accurately inferences can be made about the variable measured in a particular population (Streiner & Norman, 2008). Instruments used to measure an attribute in one population may not be considered scientifically useful for another population. For example, two instruments that were not designed for cancer patients but were seen as potentially useful for that population have been tested in this RFE (Davies, 2013; Yackzan, 2017). One of the studies is described in **BOX 5-2**.

Modify an Existing Instrument

Modify existing
instrument

There are many reasons for modifying an instrument that has been rigorously tested but does not fit the purpose of a study. Some items may not apply to the sample, the scale may not be appropriate, and scoring may not fit the projected analysis of data.

BOX 5-2 Susan Yackzan, RN, MSN, PhD, APRN, AOCN: Assessment of Anxiety Among Women with Breast Cancer: Using the DASS

Susan, a research consultant, examined the reliability and validity of a measure of anxiety, the Distress Anxiety Stress Scale (DASS), in a population of women who may experience anxiety but are not systematically assessed for that specific affective response. Women who are asked to return for a diagnostic mammogram after a false-positive mammogram have reported experiencing anxiety. Methods used to assess anxiety in this population have been varied. A number of standardized tests, single questions, and visual analogue scales have been used. The DASS is a well-established, psychometrically sound instrument used to assess anxiety among adults. Susan wanted to see if the DASS would be reliable and valid with women who were recalled for a false-positive mammogram. She used a large data set (N=2,672) from a study of women undergoing a diagnostic mammogram and calculated statistics that would evaluate reliability (internal consistency: alpha coefficient and Spearman Brown coefficient) and construct validity (hypothesis testing and principal component analysis). Outcomes suggest that the DASS anxiety subscale is a reliable and valid measure of anxiety among women undergoing a diagnostic mammogram.

For example, some of the items on a nurse retention questionnaire developed 20 years ago may be appropriate, but, given changes in nursing over time, others would not be relevant. Important issues related to the profession have been resolved and would no longer be relevant.

A study in the design phase in this RFE has required investigators to modify a well-known instrument (see **BOX 5-3**).

 BOX 5-3 Jeri Hahn, RN, ADN: The Impact of Water Therapy on Central Nervous System, Metabolic, Vasomotor, Respiratory, and Gastrointestinal Disturbances Among Neonatal Abstinence Syndrome (NAS) Babies

Jeri designed a study to examine the effect of immersing NAS babies in water to improve their well-being their first weeks of life. Born to drug-addicted mothers, these infants experience central nervous system irritability, gastrointestinal distress, excessive high-pitched crying, sleeplessness, poor feeding, and autonomic over-reactivity. Following an extensive review of the literature, the Modified Finnegan Neonatal Abstinence Score Sheet (Finnegan, 1990) was identified as a possible measure for this study. Using this scale as a foundation, an assessment of these variables was designed. A group of nurses who care for NAS babies examined each item on the Finnegan Scale, adopted some of the underlying concepts, and added items of particular interest to them. The Neonatal Abstinence Scale is the result of their work.

Develop an Instrument

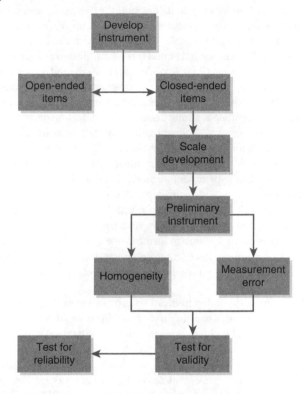

As mentioned previously, assisting caregivers to measure the variables they want to examine is a major component of the role of research consultants in this RFE. Once it is apparent that a measurement tool is not available, the process of developing an instrument that will meet caregivers' goals begins. One approach to developing items for an instrument is to identify basic concepts that need to be included. For example, in a study designed to evaluate caregivers' perceptions of the value of a "huddle" process, timeliness, satisfaction, and information sharing were important concepts to examine (Melton et al., 2017). Items were then based on those concepts. Another approach to item formation was used in a study designed to predict dysphagia among adult patients diagnosed with pneumonia (Groppo-Lawless, Bugajski, & Davies, 2018). The investigator conducted a retrospective chart review of these patients. She developed a list of symptoms taken from the literature regarding the development of dysphagia in this population and assessed their prevalence in the chart review. The most prevalent symptoms were used to develop her instrument.

For purposes of this chapter, the term *item* refers to both requests for information on questionnaires that are not written in the form of a question and questions. For example, the following request is a statement, not a question: "I am satisfied with my position" (to which someone could select either yes or no as a response). That same idea could be phrased as "Are you satisfied with your position?" Both questions and statements (items) are used on questionnaires depending on the audience and the purpose.

Open-Ended Items

Open-ended and closed-ended questions constitute the two major categories of items to consider when developing an instrument. Open-ended items are frequently designed to request an in-depth description of a variable. For example, two medical imaging technologists in this RFE designed 17 closed-ended items (three subscales) to assess their colleagues' satisfaction with their profession (Fultz & Walker, 2017). At the end of their questionnaire, they asked participants to comment on their satisfaction with their positions. Eighteen participants (30.5%) responded. Three themes consistent with the closed-ended items were derived from the comments: strong desire for competent management/leadership, good communication/teamwork, and recognition of staff for good work.

Because responses to open-ended questions are less limiting than closed-ended questions, they can provide a depth of information that adds to or affirms other findings. These responses can supplement numerical data and broaden the scope of the study topic. In addition to providing in-depth descriptions of variables, open-ended questions can simply ask individuals for a numerical response to requests for age, timing of a particular event, or frequency of an occurrence. In this case, numbers rather than words are retrieved. In addition to forming open-ended questions, investigators may simply add a Comments section at the conclusion of their questionnaire, the assumption being that participants will make comments related to the topic under investigation.

When including open-ended items in an instrument, it is important to provide sufficient space for the participant to answer. Asking an individual to respond to a question that might provoke a long response, such as "What would you like to change in your work environment?," is frustrating to the respondent if there is not enough space to provide a response. In addition, given limited space, investigators may not be able to read what is written. Depending on the area of investigation, providing an additional page for respondents may be a good idea. In this RFE, studies have used up to 1.5 pages of space for comments.

Given that asking respondents to write a response to a question takes more time and energy than checking a box for a closed-ended item, the number of comments returned may be less than desired. Attending to potential motivation for individuals to respond to a request for writing comments is important. In addition, providing a place that is comfortable for participants to respond to questionnaires may be helpful. If an area is not particularly interesting to participants, few comments or answers to open-ended questions may be written.

Personal issues, such as work satisfaction, often motivate participants to spend time writing lengthy comments. For example, 279 nurses (34.7% response rate) completed a nurse-retention questionnaire in this RFE (Bugajski et al., 2017). Nurses seemed extremely interested in participating in a study that related to their careers. One hundred ten nurses (39% response rate) wrote comments following the closed-ended items. This response rate suggests that participants were interested in factors that could improve their satisfaction with work.

In order to have a meaningful response rate when participants are asked to complete open-ended questions, investigators need to use them sparingly. Making careful decisions regarding the importance of responses to open-ended questions to the overall goal of the study is recommended (Dillman, Smyth, & Christian, 2009). In addition, providing clear directions for providing responses to open-ended questions may result in retrieving useful data.

Closed-Ended Items

Closed-ended items are limited as compared to open-ended questions because they require a fixed response. The advantage in closed-ended items is that responses are usually numerical. Statistical analyses can be conducted that permit conclusions not available from data retrieved from open-ended questions. For example, the nurse retention questionnaire developed in this RFE (Lengerich et al., 2017) contains 12 items (3 subscales). Statistical analyses were performed that enable investigators to establish content validity, identify major components of the scale (nursing practice, management, and staffing), and provide an assessment of reliability.

When developing closed-ended items, it is important to include all reasonable options reflecting the variable of interest. In order to better understand a variable, a broad, in-depth representation of all possible items is ideal. In addition, items need to be mutually exclusive. Only one idea can be assessed in one item. For example, items for the medical imaging technologists' job satisfaction questionnaire (Fultz & Walker, 2018) addressed leadership and communication. If an item reflecting those ideas stated, "Leadership and communication are important to job satisfaction," the importance of leadership versus communication would not be apparent. In the questionnaire, these two ideas, leadership and communication, are addressed in separate items.

Items also need to be developed that clearly apply to targeted respondents. A questionnaire designed to assess the birth experience of women having their first child is probably not suitable for use with mothers of several children. Accuracy in terms of information within the item is also essential. Respondents cannot provide useful information if what they are given is not accurate. A simple, straightforward expression of an item probably produces the best results. Specific, concrete terms may be helpful in guiding respondents to provide meaningful responses. In relation to words used, a common recommendation is to keep items at the reading level of a 12-year-old child. The length of items is another important consideration. Items need to convey the desired idea and also be as short as possible. Validity, or how accurately an instrument measures what it is supposed to measure, tends to decrease as the number of items increases (Norman & Streiner, 2009).

With a goal of participants completing a questionnaire accurately and completely, directions regarding how respondents should respond to the questionnaire need to be clear and succinct. When total scores are necessary to interpret the outcome of the questionnaire, respondents should be encouraged in the directions to answer each item (Dillman, Smyth, & Christian, 2009). Visually, items need to be spaced so that participants can easily determine the beginning and ending of each item. An example of a study that used an investigator-designed questionnaire is described in **BOX 5-4**.

 BOX 5-4 Kim Kjelland, APRN, MSN, PNP-BC: The Best for Baby Card: An Evaluation of Factors That Influence Women's Decisions to Breastfeed

Kim was concerned regarding the decreasing number of women breastfeeding their infants during their hospital stay. She designed a study to test the effect of an intervention (the Best for Baby Card) as well as identify those factors that may make a difference in women's decisions to breastfeed. She worked with a research consultant to design a questionnaire reflecting those factors found in the literature that were believed to influence women's

(continues)

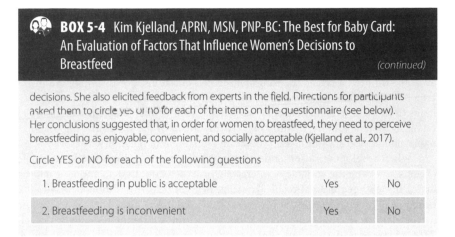

(continued)

decisions. She also elicited feedback from experts in the field. Directions for participants asked them to circle yes or no for each of the items on the questionnaire (see below). Her conclusions suggested that, in order for women to breastfeed, they need to perceive breastfeeding as enjoyable, convenient, and socially acceptable (Kjelland et al., 2017).

Circle YES or NO for each of the following questions

1. Breastfeeding in public is acceptable	Yes	No
2. Breastfeeding is inconvenient	Yes	No

Scale Development

How numbers are assigned to items depends on how many categories of responses are appropriate. The number of categories selected determines the level of measurement, and the level of measurement influences decisions related to statistical analysis. The goal of assigning numbers is to provide sufficient categories for the respondent to make a reasonable choice. A reasonable choice suggests that the categories are neither too far apart nor too close. Numerical responses to items can result in one of four different levels of measurement: nominal, ordinal, interval, and ratio. Nominal level of measurement occurs when numbers assigned to the attribute under investigation represent mutually exclusive categories. At this level, categories cannot be ordered or ranked in any way; they are used for labeling purposes only. For example, categorizing participants as "does smoke" and "does not smoke" describes a quality rather than a quantity. Nominal data were analyzed in the study described in **BOX 5-5**.

When numbers assigned to variables are rank ordered, an ordinal level of measurement results. Using an ordinal level of measurement, the variable measured is separated according to the amount of the variable present. This ordering, however, does not suggest that intervals between scale categories are equal. Scaling in this manner simply means that the second rank has more of the variable assessed than the first. For example, ranking participants one to three as to their ability to manage a chronic condition (one = difficulty managing condition, two = somewhat comfortable managing condition, three = very comfortable managing condition) results in ordinal level data. A numerical continuum is not reflected in the scale.

Unlike the ordinal level of measurement, the interval level assumes an equal space between each number: The amount of the variable between one and two is the same as the amount between two and three. Amounts of the variable are spread equally over the length of the scale (Walt, Strickland, & Lenz, 2010). The Likert scale is an example of a scaling approach that can result in an interval level of measurement. It is often used to assess agreement or disagreement with a component of the variable measured. However, many other descriptors, in addition to agreement and disagreement, may be used (Norman & Streiner, 2009).

While interval measurement requires an assumption that equal spaces exist between each scale number, there is no zero point—for example, there is no zero point

BOX 5-5 Debra Lewis, RN, BSN: The Effect of Three Nursing Interventions on Thermoregulation in Low-Birthweight Infants

Debra evaluated the effect of occlusive wrap, chemical mattress, and regulation of room temperature on thermoregulation among low-birthweight infants (N=67). Interventions were applied one at a time and together. The research team consisted of staff nurses, a neonatologist, a unit educator, an outcomes coordinator, and a research consultant. As a part of the study, normal versus abnormal temperatures were determined. Given that temperature data were nominal, chi-squares (nonparametric tests) were calculated. Results provided initial support for the use of these three interventions (Lewis, Sanders, & Brockopp, 2011).

for well-being or satisfaction. The ratio level of measurement is similar to interval level, but with the addition of a zero point. Money is an example of a variable that could be measured using a ratio level of measurement because it is possible to have no money. If you have zero money, the implication is the absence of money.

Deciding how many categories a scale will have can be a challenge. If there are too many categories, the difference between each category is so small it may be meaningless. While the investigator's judgment plays an important role in identifying the number of categories, there are recommended guidelines. If the questionnaire is assessing both the direction and extent of an attribute, five or seven categories are recommended—for example, when respondents are asked to assess their satisfaction with their role as well as the extent of their satisfaction. When the goal is to assess the extent of an attribute only (i.e., not important, somewhat important, very important, extremely important), four or five categories are suggested. Adding more scale points beyond this adds modest increases in reliability and validity (Dillman, Smyth, & Christian, 2009).

Visual analogue scales (VAS) are also used in healthcare research to assess variables of interest. Data analyzed using these scales are often considered interval. Both clinically and when conducting research, scales of 1 to 5 or 1 to 10 are frequently used to measure the extent of pain an individual is experiencing. Participants in a study may be given a piece of paper and asked to circle a number from 1 to 10 or make a mark on a line of specified length. One of the difficulties when using a VAS is that only one aspect of the experience is assessed. Particularly in the measurement of pain, additional information regarding the individual's experience with pain may be necessary in order to obtain meaningful information related to care.

As previously mentioned, the importance of understanding levels of measurement in relation to the scale selected to assess a variable is related to the statistical analysis of data retrieved. The scale assigned to evaluate a variable of interest guides the selection of a statistical test. There is a conservative approach to making decisions regarding what statistical test should be used as well as a more pragmatic approach. Both agree that when either nominal or ordinal levels of measurement are used, a nonparametric statistical test is required (e.g., chi square).

There is, however, controversy regarding which statistical test should be used when the attribute is measured on a continuum. For example, use of a Likert scale (i.e., 1 = strongly disagree, 2 = disagree, 3 = agree, 4 = strongly agree) suggests that the variable of interest can be assessed using continuous numbers. Items in the

Scales of Psychological Well-Being (Ryff, 1989) used in a study at this RFE to assess the well-being of women diagnosed with breast cancer pre- and post diagnosis (Lengerich et al., 2018) are measured using a Likert scale. Using this scale, respondents circle a number, from one to six, to reflect their degree of agreement with the item. A conservative choice of statistical tests requires assurance that the difference between numbers on the scale reflects actual differences in the well-being of each participant. If that equal difference is affirmed, parametric statistics can be used (e.g., t test.) The practical approach recommends minimizing the emphasis on the differences between numbers on the scale and focusing more on the nature of the research question posed (Waltz, Strickland, & Lenz, 2010).

Preliminary Instrument

Following the construction of items and identification of a scale, other criteria used to assess the effectiveness of an instrument can be addressed. Homogeneity refers to how similarly items measure the same variable. Moderate similarity is considered appropriate. There are also a number of potential errors of measurement. These criteria need to be considered when developing an instrument.

Testing Items for Homogeneity

One of the goals in constructing items for a questionnaire is to include items that will assess different aspects of the same variable. The questionnaire should not, however, include items that have little relationship to the area of interest; for example, if a questionnaire is assessing job satisfaction, items should not be measuring job competence. In order to assess how closely items are related one to another, an investigator can compute a correlation coefficient (Pearson product moment correlation). This coefficient is calculated by comparing the score of each item with the total score of the instrument. The score for each item must be removed prior to calculating the coefficient so that the item is not correlated with itself. Each item should be moderately correlated with the total score (above 0.20) or discarded (Norman & Streiner, 2009).

Criteria for Evaluating the Scientific Usefulness of Measures: Errors

When initiating the development of an instrument, it is important to consider a set of criteria for evaluating the scientific usefulness of measures. These criteria are termed errors of measurement. While there are no perfect measures, the goal of developing a measure is to avoid errors as much as possible. However, errors can occur regardless of the stringent testing of a given measure. Even those instruments designed to measure variables with a high degree of precision can fail in terms of providing accurate information.

Five errors are commonly thought to produce inaccurate information if they are present during the assessment process. Situational contaminants include conditions that may influence the outcome of the measure. For example, asking a teenager to respond to a set of questions with a parent present may modify their responses. Response set bias occurs when individuals tend to respond in a specific fashion regardless of the topic under consideration. They may, for example, answer questions in the extreme even if that does not accurately represent their opinion. Transitory personal factors refer to states of mind that inhibit an accurate response to a question—respondents may be tired or upset over a life situation. Administration variations can influence participants' responses to items in terms of time taken to respond or concentration on the task at hand. For example, some questionnaires may be given to participants in a face-to-face situation while others are sent to individuals at their homes. Those who respond at home may be able to take more time and expend more energy completing the questionnaire. Item sampling can be another source of measurement error. If a questionnaire is too long, individuals may be reluctant to take the time to complete all items; if it is too short, important issues may not be addressed and accurate information not revealed. While investigators try to consider and minimize these errors of measurement, they inevitably will occur (Polit & Hungler, 2006).

For example, two studies of infants—one that assessed infant well-being in the NICU (Stoltz et al., 2014) and another that examined the effect of massage on babies suffering from NAS (Hahn et al., 2015)—could have been subject to errors of measurement. Assessing well-being of these neonates could have been influenced by parent involvement (situational contaminants). The effect of massage on NAS babies could have been impacted by mothers' emotional status given their concerns for their infants (transitory personal factors). As previously mentioned, in most measurement situations, errors of some kind will, in all likelihood, exist. Even so, information retrieved from studies can be meaningful in relation to changing practice.

Criteria for Assessing Measures: Validity

Validity, when used to describe a measure, refers to the ability of that measure to assess what it was intended to assess. Validity does not refer to a given instrument but to the use of that instrument to meet a goal within a specific population (Streiner & Norman, 2009). Face validity, content validity, construct validity, and criterion validity are criteria related to the scientific usefulness of a measure. Face validity refers to whether or not the instrument appears to measure the variable of interest. The other forms of validity are more important when judging the usefulness of a particular instrument in retrieving meaningful data.

Content Validity. Content validity refers to how well items in a given measure represent all possible items related to the variable of interest. For example, if an investigator was interested in developing an instrument to measure depression, it would be important for each item on the instrument to reflect the different aspects of depression. Given that depression includes affective and physical symptoms, the instrument should include items that address both areas. For example, the instrument may have one item about physical symptoms, such as "I have little energy," as well as affective symptoms, such as "I feel blue." Nunnally (1978) provides two standards for ensuring content validity. The first refers to the importance of representing all possible aspects of the variable studied, while the second is selecting a reasonable approach to identifying items.

Content validity is relevant for measures that assess affect, cognition, and physiological change. For example, measuring parents' perception of infant well-being in a NICU can involve affect or feelings (Stoltz et al., 2014). Parents assessed the comfort level of their vulnerable infants, and so clearly some emotion could have been involved in their assessment. The Brockopp Warden Pain Knowledge Questionnaire assesses nurses' knowledge of pain management. Experts in the area of pain management reviewed the items for content validity. Content validity was assessed in Honaker and colleagues' (2014) study examining the existence and progress of deep-tissue injuries. In this study, the authors developed a risk assessment for suspected deep-tissue injury severity and progression. To establish validity for this instrument, the investigators asked for feedback from a panel of experts in this field. The instrument was then revised based on their expertise.

Selecting items that are truly representative of all possible items related to a given concept is a difficult task. Random sampling of a long list of possible items is one method for developing an instrument (Waltz, Strickland, & Lentz, 2010). Literature reviews and expert opinion are two additional methods generally used in this RFE. Asking a panel of experts to suggest and review content relevant for the development of a specific instrument is a frequently used strategy. The responses of an expert panel can be analyzed statistically to determine degree of agreement among experts and can be further analyzed to support a given instrument's content validity.

In addition, the type of individual (e.g., inpatient) who will respond to an instrument may contribute to the development of items. For example, a study (Corley et al., 2014) designed to predict the likelihood of inpatients' falling used data from inpatients who had fallen to construct the instrument. Another example of using experts plus the literature to develop items is described in **BOX 5-6**.

Testing for content validity occurs after the initial development of an instrument. Once items have been identified, a content validity index (CVI) can be calculated. Experts rate each item for relevance to the topic of interest on a one to four scale (a score of one suggests that the item is not relevant, while four rates the item as relevant). The index reflects the percentage of total item ratings at either three or four. A percentage of 80 or above is considered good content validity. Modifications can be made to the instrument based on the CVI until a percentage of 80 or above is reached.

Waltz, Strickland, and Lentz (2010) recommend calculating an alpha coefficient when more than two experts are involved in rating an instrument. An alpha coefficient

 BOX 5-6 Alex Lengerich, MS, EdS: The Baptist Health Nurse Retention Questionnaire—A Methodological Study, Part 1

Nurse retention in the hospital setting is a concern across the United States. Alex was asked to lead a study investigating those factors that could lead to a high rate of retention for hospital-based nurses. A comprehensive review of the literature revealed a number of questionnaires focused solely on work environment. More broadly based assessments were more than 10 years old. Fifteen articles describing retention issues were reviewed and possible factors that could influence retention identified. A group of nurse administrators, clinical nurses, and research consultants gathered to review and revise proposed factors. Following the selection of 12 items, content validity was evaluated using a content validity index. The resulting questionnaire was published (Lengerich et al., 2017).

BOX 5-7 Heather Bradley, MSN, RN: Evaluating Preceptors— A Methodological Study

Given changes in the hospital setting related to higher patient acuity and resulting additional expectations of nurses, Heather, a nurse educator, was concerned about the difficulties new graduates may have transitioning from school to practice. Preceptors of new graduates are key to making this transition successful. Heather's goal was to develop a valid, reliable, and clinically useful instrument that would evaluate the performance and proficiency of preceptors. A multisite (four hospitals) study was proposed and funded by the Association for Nursing Professional Development. The instrument was designed for new graduates and administrators to assess preceptors. Preceptors would also use the instrument to conduct a self-evaluation. Following a comprehensive review of the literature, experts were asked to review and provide feedback on potential items for the questionnaire. Nurse experts (N=12) across four hospitals participated in establishing content validity. A CVI was calculated for each of 28 items with a range of 0.92 to 1.00. Her study was published (Bradley et al., 2015), and 25 educators at other hospitals and graduate nursing students across the United States have asked to use the instrument. An example of items follows.

During orientation, my preceptor. . .

	Strongly Disagree	Disagree	Agree	Strongly Agree
1. Helped me to develop confidence in my nursing role				
2. Assessed my learning needs				
3. Built on my previous experience				
4. Collaborated with me to design learning goals				

reflects the consistency of responses across experts. Similar to the CVI, the higher the number between 0 and 1, the greater the agreement that items are relevant. An example of the use of the CVI is presented in **BOX 5-7**.

Construct Validity. In addition to content validity, construct validity is an important criterion to address when developing an instrument. Construct validity refers to the extent to which items included in the instrument are consistent with the variable measured. Establishing construct validity is more difficult for theoretical constructs than concrete concepts. A conceptual framework can be helpful when trying to establish construct validity. For example, the development of Ryff's Scales of Psychological Well-Being (Ryff, 1989) came from a theoretical perspective that well-being supports a positive affective state rather than the absence of negative affect. Given that theoretical perspective, items could be constructed to reflect that particular way of thinking about well-being.

Both logic and conducting specific tests contribute to the assessment of construct validity. If study variables are more subjective than objective, judgment will be more likely to play a role in assessing construct validity. Specific approaches for testing construct validity include comparing the results of an existing measure of the same construct with the newly designed measure, hypothesis testing of an intervention on scores retrieved, and using statistical tests such as factor analysis (Waltz, Strickland, & Lenz, 2010).

Comparison of Measures. Frequently, measures of a construct that an investigator wants to examine do not exist. However, investigators may want to develop a questionnaire even though one is available. For example, the Baptist Health High Risk Falls Assessment (BHHRFA; Corley et al., 2014) requires a nurse to respond to 16 items. If someone wanted to develop a shorter assessment and wanted to assess construct validity, he or she might compare the scores with those of the BHHFRA. Differences in mean scores could be calculated to ascertain whether or not the same attributes were measured.

Hypothesis Testing. Hypothesis testing requires investigators to identify one or more hypotheses from the conceptual framework that provides the foundation for the variable of interest. For example, the concept of "nurse position" as it relates to nurse retention suggests that nurses in a hospital setting choose to remain in their positions if the overall patient care provided is good to excellent (Bugajski et al., 2017). The hypothesis that nurse satisfaction will be greater on units that provide good to excellent care could be tested. To test this hypothesis, the investigator would collect data on nurse satisfaction and patient care. If a strong relationship existed between these two variables, there is evidence for construct validity.

Statistical Tests to Assess Construct Validity. Investigators who design an instrument to reflect differing dimensions or components of a variable can use statistical tests to evaluate construct validity. Factor analysis is a process that enables investigators to discover major components or subscales within their list of items. Initially, the instrument is given to a large representative sample of participants. Complex analyses follow that involve two phases. The goal of these phases is to group highly interrelated items together. The first phase involves identifying factors from a correlation matrix. The second phase uses factor rotation to better understand which items should be subsumed under each factor. In-depth explanations of these analyses are readily available in measurement texts (Norman & Streiner, 2009; Waltz, Strickland, & Lenz, 2010). An example of one type of factor analysis used in the nurse retention study conducted in this RFE is presented in **BOX 5-8**.

Criterion-Related Validity. Criterion-related validity refers to the extent an instrument measures an individual's position on a variable that differs from the one being measured. There are two kinds of criterion-related validity: predictive and concurrent. Timing is the difference in these two kinds of criterion-related validity. Predictive validity is future oriented. For example, if nurses are given a questionnaire that assesses their knowledge of effective pain management, and their patients are

> **BOX 5-8** Alex Lengerich, MS, EdS: The Baptist Health Nurse Retention Questionnaire (BHNRQ)—A Methodological Study, Part 1 (Continued)
>
> Validity and reliability were tested following the development of the BHNRQ (Lengerich et al., 2017). Two hundred seventy-nine (34.7% response rate) nurses completed the questionnaire. Content validity was tested using a CVI. Based on their expertise as clinicians, unit managers selected five clinical nurses to serve as content experts. Each of these nurses completed a questionnaire asking them to rate the relevance of each item included on the BHNRQ. Each item was scored on a four-point Likert scale ranging from one (not relevant) to four (highly relevant). The number of responses of either "quite relevant" or "highly relevant" was added and divided by the total number of nurses who responded to the questionnaire. All items were considered "highly relevant," with CVI scores ranging from 0.80 to 1.00. To test predictive validity, a principal components analysis (PCA; a type of factor analysis) was conducted. Three factors were identified: nursing practice, management, and staffing. Ten nurses were involved in testing reliability (consistency over time) of the instrument. These individuals responded to the questionnaire on two occasions, 2 weeks apart. Because the sample size did not reach 300 (the suggested sample size in order to calculate an alpha coefficient), reliability in the form of internal consistency was not calculated.

assessed as having less pain at some later time, that instrument could be said to have predictive validity. Concurrent validity reflects how well an instrument can identify individuals who fall into a particular category—for example, does nursing students' performance on a test focused on drug calculation suggest that they are accurate when giving drugs?

Sensitivity and Specificity

Calculations of sensitivity and specificity can provide an assessment of the predictive validity of an instrument. Sensitivity refers to the percentage of cases that can be classified as accurately representing the variable measured (true positives). For example, if an investigator is interested in developing an instrument that measures knowledge level of new nurse graduates prior to graduation as a predictor of licensure examination pass rates, a calculation of sensitivity would show the percentage that would pass. Specificity (calculation of sensitivity showing percentage passing) represents the percentage of cases wherein knowledge level does not predict passing the examination (true negatives).

Diagnostic Odds Ratio

The diagnostic odds ratio (DOR) is a statistical test that is often performed in addition to sensitivity and specificity. This ratio is a single indicator of an instrument's performance. In the example above, the DOR is the ratio of the odds of nurses passing the exam to the odds of nurses failing the exam. The range of possible scores is zero to infinity. In general, useful tests have a DOR greater than 1 (Pallant, 2007).

The high-risk falls assessment developed in this RFE was assessed for predictive validity. The example is presented in **BOX 5-9**.

BOX 5-9 Donna Corley, RN, MSN, PhD: The Baptist Health High Risk Falls
Assessment: A Methodological Study

Accidental falls in an acute care setting can result in serious injuries. Given this
fact, a group of nurses along with research consultants initiated a 5-year project
to develop an instrument that could predict those adult inpatients who would
be at high risk for falling (Corley et al., 2014). Following a two-phase process for
developing the questionnaire (BHHFRA), 241,599 assessments at four hospitals
were collected. Sensitivity of the instrument across hospitals was 0.70, and
specificity was 0.66. The DOR was 4.73. Given the difficulty to date in predicting
inpatients who might fall, this assessment is recommended for use based on its
psychometric properties.

Reliability

The reliability of a measure refers to the degree that it consistently assesses the variable
of interest. Assessments of consistency over time, internal consistency, parallel form
equivalence, and interrater agreement are methods for testing the reliability of an
instrument. Both reliability and validity are important criteria when developing an
instrument, and they are not completely independent of each other. A measure of an
attribute that is not reliable cannot be valid, and an instrument that appears to be valid
cannot adequately assess the attribute of interest if results are erratic or inaccurate.
However, a measure can be reliable and not valid—consistency can exist without the
instrument actually assessing what it is purported to measure.

Consistency over Time

Stability of an instrument over time is an important criterion when assessing reliability.
If the results of a measure, using the same participants, change over a brief period of
time, trust in results diminishes. A test–retest approach provides evidence regarding
the stability of the measure. Using this approach, the instrument is given to the same
individuals on two occasions. There are differing views on how many individuals
should be involved; recommendations include calculating a power analysis prior to
collecting data (Paiva et al., 2017) or asking five times the number of individuals as
there are items to respond (Park et al., 2017).

The designated time period between administering the first and second test is
based on the purpose of the instrument. The goal in testing consistency over time is
for the same participants to respond to the measure over a time period that prevents
them from simply remembering the items on the instrument and responding from
memory, yet not so long that change could have occurred due to life circumstances.

For example, the nurse retention questionnaire developed in this RFE (Lengerich
et al., 2017) has as an item "Quality care is provided." Possible responses are "Rarely
exists," "Exists some of the time," and "Exists most of the time." A respondent asked to
complete the questionnaire within a few days of the first administration may circle the
same response based on remembering the item. For these kinds of items, a 10-day to
2-week period between administrations is recommended. In other situations, a shorter
time period may be appropriate. For example, physical therapists may see change in a

BOX 5-10 Claire Davies, PT, PhD, CLT-LANA: Test–Retest and Internal Consistency of the Disability of Arm, Shoulder, and Hand (DASH) Outcome Measure in Assessing Functional Status Among Breast Cancer Survivors

Claire, an expert in the area of lymphedema in breast cancer survivors, was interested in assessing the consistency over time of the DASH for use with this population (Davies, 2013). Outpatients (N=19) were asked to respond to the instrument on two occasions separated by 2 to 3 hours. This time period was chosen so that symptom fluctuation would not influence the outcome of the assessment. A reliability coefficient (intraclass correlation) of 0.97 was determined.

patient's functional status within hours. Testing a functional status scale for consistency over time may require investigators to give the second test within one or two hours.

Statistical analyses used to indicate how closely responses to the first administration of the measure relate to responses to the second administration include Pearson Product Moment (Pearson's r) correlations and intraclass correlations. Correlations describe the strength of the coefficient ranging from -1 to 1. A probability value or confidence interval is also reported. These values convey how likely the outcome is repeatable. An example of a study that tested consistency over time is presented in **BOX 5-10**.

Internal Consistency. Internal consistency refers to the extent to which individuals respond to items across the instrument in the same way. For example, if job satisfaction is the focus of a questionnaire, items related to dietary preferences would probably not be appropriate. Similar to test–retest reliability, a correlation coefficient (alpha coefficient) is calculated to determine internal consistency. The coefficient ranges from 0 to 1: 0.70 is considered, in most instances, to show an acceptable level of internal consistency. When calculating an alpha coefficient, a sample size of 300 is recommended (Yurdugul, 2008). Given this recommendation, newly developed instruments may not have been tested on a sample that large, and, as a result, internal consistency coefficients are not reported.

Parallel Form Equivalence. When two forms of an instrument can be developed, a parallel form procedure can be used to evaluate reliability. Both forms are given to the same group of individuals, and differences between outcomes are assessed. If a significant difference does not exist and variances are similar, then good reliability is assumed (Waltz, Strickland, & Lenz, 2010).

Interrater Reliability. Testing for interrater reliability occurs when more than one individual uses the same instrument at the same time to rate a specific attribute of interest. For example, if two nurses, independently and at the same time, use an instrument to assess symptom behaviors among infants diagnosed with NAS, their responses can be analyzed to determine interrater reliability of the instrument. A reliability coefficient can be calculated to demonstrate the similarity of responses. Another approach to analysis, the calculation of percent agreement (Po) and kappa (K) is also suggested (Waltz, Strickland, & Lenz, 2010). An example of a study that includes the calculation of interrater reliability is presented in **BOX 5-11**.

BOX 5-11 Jeremy Honaker, RN, BSN, CWOCN: Development and Psychometric Testing of the Honaker Suspected Deep-Tissue Injury Severity Scale (HSDTISS)

Jeremy's study was designed to develop an instrument that would assess the severity of a suspected deep-tissue injury as well as the progression of these injuries (Honaker, Brockopp, & Moe, 2014). Following the initial development of the HSDTISS, it was reviewed for content validity by 10 experts in the area of wound healing. Changes were made based on their review. Ease of use was evaluated by 10 clinical nurses representing differing areas of patient care. Results of caregivers' assessments indicated that the instrument was easy to use, required minimal time to complete, and could effectively guide clinical interventions; thus, no changes were made. Finally, interrater reliability was addressed. Twenty-one clinicians (6 physical therapists and 15 nurses) used the instrument to rate photographs of injuries. An intraclass correlation coefficient was calculated ($r = 0.997$, $p < 0.001$) showing excellent correlation among reviewers.

Administer the Instrument

Administer
instrument

Once an instrument is developed, there are a number of approaches that can be used to collect data. Cost, desired number of responses, and how items are designed can influence the approach used. Cost may be a more important issue for investigators in community hospitals as opposed to university associated medical centers. Given the resources generally available at medical centers, federal and regional grants are often options that are not as accessible to investigators at community hospitals. Funds awarded in this RFE over a 9-year period ($154,000; 17 projects) have come largely from vendors or professional organizations. Although most of the grants have been small (less than $20,000), they have covered the cost of data collectors and individuals to input data. Both activities can be time consuming and therefore costly.

The number of responses desired is dependent on the design of the study. The goal is to reach a specific number of participants as designated by a power analysis, or in some cases simply reach as many participants as possible. Responses to quantitative self-reports can be accessed face-to-face at one point in time or face-to-face at several data collection points. Responses can also be retrieved using the telephone, the Internet, and mailings. When using mailed questionnaires, including a self-addressed stamped envelope will ensure a greater response rate.

The goal of collecting information about a specific variable is to reach as representative a sample of the population of interest as possible. Response rates provide information regarding how well participants represent the chosen sample. Uncertainty related to the accuracy of response rates is common. The method of data collection can impact the degree of certainty related to a given response rate. For example, there may be some uncertainty as to whether or not a questionnaire posted on the Internet has reached the participant; when phones are used, they may be disconnected or inoperable; and mailed questionnaires may get lost. When compared to other data-collection approaches, a face-to-face approach occurring on one occasion probably results in the highest response rate.

Face-to-face encounters usually involve a trained individual interacting with participants as they complete an instrument or answer questions verbally. Compliance is generally very good as participants are comfortable, can ask questions if confused, and are focused on the task. In addition, from an investigator's point of view, face-to-face encounters permit clear identification of who is participating. Face-to-face encounters can occur on one or more occasion, depending on the design of the study. When compared to other data collection approaches, a face-to-face approach occurring on one occasion probably results in the highest response rate. Higher cost may be a disadvantage of face-to-face encounters. If an individual is asking questions of participants, training is most likely involved. In addition, personnel costs increase when one individual needs to spend time with each participant.

Telephone interviews are another option for collecting data. Similar to face-to-face encounters, interviewers need training to ensure consistency of data collection. In addition, although an increasing number of individuals in the United States have ready access to a cell phone, problems have arisen in this RFE related to potential participants for a study not having access to a phone. Another issue to consider, if planning to conduct telephone interviews, is the possibility that someone else in the household might prompt the participant. Advantages of both face-to-face encounters and telephone calls include a reduction in the number of missed items, the fact that open-ended questions can be included, and that the data collector will know if the participant has difficulty understanding the items.

The Internet can also be a medium for collecting data. In many instances, use of a computer has replaced the use of paper and pencil tests. Advantages include less time involved, as the instrument can be administered to a number of people simultaneously; reduction in transcription errors; and decreased cost. One disadvantage is that paper and pencil instruments allow participants to view the entire questionnaire at once and review their response to prior items, while Internet-based questionnaires may not permit participants to do the same.

Mailed questionnaires can be coordinated by one individual, which can diminish cost related to personnel and investigators' time. Although mailing questionnaires is a fairly simple approach to collecting data, questions arise during the process. If not returned, the investigator may wonder if the envelope reached the appropriate individual. Reminders need to be sent out, and, because there is no interaction between data collector and participant, responses to some of the items are frequently missed.

Strategies used to encourage a high response rate for all methods used include the following: including a clear, brief, and encouraging cover letter; letting participants know that a questionnaire is coming to them; giving a token of appreciation; ensuring anonymity; using a participant's name and address rather than "occupant"; and enclosing a self-addressed stamped envelope for return of the information. Cover letters can provide the reason for the study and therefore encourage individuals to participate. Giving potential participants warning that a questionnaire is coming diminishes the likelihood that the envelope will be discarded. Even a small token of appreciation has been found to increase response rate. Ensuring anonymity is key to individuals' comfort in responding to questions asked. When the address is to the "occupant" rather than an individual, the questionnaire is more likely to be discarded. Finally, enclosing a self-addressed stamped return envelope is key to getting individuals to respond (Streiner & Norman, 2009).

A sample cover letter is presented in **EXHIBIT 5-1**.

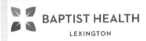

EXHIBIT 5-1 Sample Cover Letter

BAPTIST HEALTH
LEXINGTON

IRB NUMBER: BHL-16-1326
IRB APPROVAL DATE: 04/25/2016
IRB EXPIRATION DATE: 04/18/2017
PHONE: 859.260.6100

1740 Nicholasville Road   Lexington, KY 40503

You are invited to participate in a nursing research study at Baptist Health Lexington entitled "Nurse Retention: Preventing Turnover". This study will look at the factors that influence nurse retention. The information gained from this study will be used to help improve the retention of nurses.

Participation in this study involves completion of a survey that will take approximately 5-10 minutes. If you agree to participate, please complete the survey and place it in the lock box located at the Nurse's Station on your unit. <u>All responses are anonymous</u>.

Your participation or lack of participation will not change your employment at Baptist Health Lexington or the Baptist Health System. The only risk to you, if you choose to participate, is the potential loss of confidentiality. We will make every effort to prevent anyone who is not on the research team from knowing that you gave us information, or what that information contains. Any information you provide will be kept in a confidential file that only the research team can access. This study may be reviewed by the Baptist Health Lexington Institutional Review Board (IRB).

Completing this questionnaire can contribute to our knowledge about retaining nursing staff. Study results may be submitted for publication in a national journal but you will not be identified as a participant in the study. Of course, you have a choice about whether or not to complete the survey. If you do participate, you are free to skip any questions or discontinue at any time.

Thank you in advance for your anticipated participation.

Drew Bugajski, BSN, RN
Research Consultant
Nursing and Allied Health Research Office
Baptist Health Lexington
Doctoral Fellow
PhD student, University of Kentucky
Phone: 859-260-6893

Courtesy of Baptist Health Lexington

▶ Chapter Summary

The most important component of the instrument development process is clarification of the investigator's purpose in designing an instrument. If a psychometrically strong assessment of a clinically important variable is not available, investigators may design a project to develop a clinically useful instrument. Considerable rigor in terms of testing this kind of instrument is required if it is to be used across settings on a continuous basis. Development of the high-risk falls assessment in this RFE is an example of rigorous testing (Corley et al., 2014) .

Questionnaires may also be developed in order to examine a specific variable of interest. Factors related to work satisfaction (Fultz et al., 2017), breastfeeding (Kjelland et al., 2014), and hourly rounding (Bragg et al., 2016) are variables that have been studied in this RFE. Given that instruments were not available to examine these variables, questionnaires were developed. Testing of these questionnaires was less rigorous than the testing that occurred during the development of the high-risk falls assessment.

TABLE 5-1 provides information regarding the testing of five instruments developed in this RFE. The purpose of each of these instruments was to publish an assessment

TABLE 5-1 Testing of Instruments Developed for Use Across Settings

Variable of Interest	Testing That Occurred	Publication in Peer-Reviewed Journals
Risk of inpatients falling	Construct validity (using sensitivity, specificity, and DOR) Ease of use (time taken to administer)	Corley, D., Brockopp, D., McCowan, D., Merritt, S., Cobb, T., Johnson, Stout, C., Moe, K., & Hall, B. (2014). The Baptist Health High Risk Falls Assessment: A methodological study. *Journal of Nursing Administration, 44*(5), 263–269.
The severity of a suspected deep- tissue injury and determining its progression	Content validity Interrater reliability Ease of use	Honaker, J., Brockopp, D., & Moe, K. (2014). Development and psychometric testing of the Honaker suspected deep tissue injury severity scale. *Journal of Wound, Ostomy and Continence Nursing, 41*(3), 238–241.
The competency and proficiency of new graduate nurses	Content validity (calculated CVIs) Test–retest reliability Internal consistency	Bradley, H., Cantrell, D., Dollahan, K., Hall, B., Lewis, P., . . . , White, D. (2015). Evaluating preceptors: A methodological study. *Journal for Nurses in Professional Development, 31*(3), 164–169.
Factors that influence hospital-based nurses to remain in their positions	Content validity Construct validity (using factor analysis) Test–retest reliability	Lengerich, A., Bugajski, A., Marchese, M., Hall, B., Tackzan, S., Davies, C., & Brockopp, D. (2017). The Baptist Health Nurse Retention questionnaire: A methodological study. (2017). *Journal of Nursing Administration, 47*(5), 289–293.
Risk for dysphagia among patients post extubation	Content validity Construct validity (using factor analysis, sensitivity, specificity, and DOR)	Moynahan. S., Swigert, N., Steele, C., & Lengerich, A. (2018). Development of the Baptist Health dysphagia screening for patients postextubation. Manuscript submitted for publication.
Risk for dysphagia among patients with a primary diagnosis of pneumonia	Content validity Construct validity (using sensitivity, specificity, and DOR)	Groppo-Lawless, S., Bugajski, D., & Davies, C. Development of the Baptist Health dysphagia screen for patients admitted with a diagnosis of pneumonia. Manuscript submitted for publication.

TABLE 5-2 Testing of Instruments Developed to Measure an Attribute for a Specific Study

Variable of Interest	Testing That Occurred	Publication in Peer-Reviewed Journals
How types of sleep surface impact well-being among infants in the NICU—one question developed for parents to assess the infants' comfort level	No testing	Stoltz, R., Byrd, R., Hench, A., Slone, T., Brockopp, D., & Moe, K. (2014). Does the type of sleep surface influence infant well-being in the NICU? *American Journal of Maternal Child Nursing, 39*(6), 363–368.
Patients' perceptions of hourly rounding—questionnaire designed to assess perceptions	Content validity	Bugajski, A., Marchese, M., Caldwell, R., Houle, L., Thompson, R., . . . , Lengerich, A. (2016). How do patients perceive hourly rounding? *Nursing Management, 47*(11), 11–13.
Factors that influence women's decision to breastfeed	Content validity	Kjelland, K., Corley, D., Slusher, I., Moe, K., & Brockopp, D. (2014). The Best for Baby card: An evaluation of factors that influence women's decisions to breastfeed. *Newborn & Infant Nursing Reviews, 14*(1), 23–27.
Work satisfaction of medical imaging technologists	Content validity	Fultz, A., Walker, A., Lengerich, A., & Bugajski, D. (2018). Radiologic Technologists' Job Satisfaction. *Radiologic Technology, 89*(6), 536–540.

that could be used across inpatient settings. Either instruments related to the variables of interest were not available or they were not sufficiently strong in terms of validity and reliability, motivating investigators to design new assessments.

TABLE 5-2 describes instruments designed to measure a variable related to a particular area of interest. These questionnaires were not developed with a goal of recommending them for use across settings. Although testing occurred in the development of these instruments, it was not as rigorous as the testing of those instruments described in Table 5-1.

References

Agency for Healthcare Research and Quality. Preventing falls in hospitals. Retrieved from http://www.ahrq.gov/professionals/systems/hospital/fallpxtoolkit/fallpxtkover.html

Bradley, H., Cantrell, D., Dollahan, K., Hall, B., Lewis, P., Merritt, S., . . . , White, D. (2015). Evaluating preceptors: A methodological study. *Journal of Nurses Professional Development, 31*(3), 164–169. doi:10.1097/nnd.0000000000000166

Bragg, L., Bugajski, A., Marchese, M., Caldwell, R., Houle, L., Thompson, R., . . . , Lengerich, A. (2016). How do patients perceive hourly rounding? *Nursing Management, 47*(11), 11–13. doi:10.1097/01 .NUMA.0000502807.60295.c5

Brockopp, D. Y., Warden, S., Colclough, G. & Brockopp, G. (1993). Nursing knowledge: Acute postoperative pain management in the elderly. *Journal of Gerontological Nursing, 19*(11), 31–37.

Bugajski, A., Lengerich, A., McCowan, D., Merritt, S., Moe, K., Hall, B., . . . , Brockopp, D. (2017). The Baptist Health High-Risk Falls Assessment: One assessment fits all. *Journal of Nursing Care and Quality, 32*(2), 114–119. doi:10.1097/ncq.0000000000000220

Corley, D., Brockopp, D., McCowan, D., Merritt, S., Cobb, T., Johnson, B., . . . , Hall, B. (2014). The Baptist Health High Risk Falls Assessment: A methodological study. *Journal of Nursing Administration, 44*(5), 263-269.

Davies, C., & Howell, D. (2012). A qualitative study: Clinical decision making in low back pain. *Physiotherapy Theory and Practice, 28*(2), 95–107. doi:10.3109/09593985.2011.571752

Davies, C., Brockopp, D., & Moe, K. (2015). Test-retest and internal consistency of the Disability of Arm, Shoulder and Hand (DASH) outcome measure in assessing functional status among breast cancer survivors with lymphedema. *Rehabilitation Oncology, 33*(1), 28–31. doi:10.1097 /ncc.0000000000000413

Davies, C. C., Brockopp, D. Y., Moe, K., Wheeler, P., Abner, J., & Lengerich, A. (2017). Exploring the lived experience of women immediately following mastectomy: A phenomenological study. *Cancer Nursing, 40*(5), 361–368.

Dillman, D., Smyth, J., & Christian, L. (2009). *Internet, mail and mixed-mode surveys: The tailored design method.* Hoboken, NJ: John Wiley & Sons.

Finnegan, L. P. (1990). Neonatal abstinence syndrome: Assessment and pharmacotherapy. In N. Nelson, ed. *Current therapy in neonatal perinatal medicine* (2nd ed.). Toronto, Ontario: BC Decker.

Fultz, A., Walker, A., Lengerich, A., & Bugajski, D. (2018). Radiologic Technologists' Job Satisfaction, *Radiologic Technology, 89*(6), 536-540.

Groppo-Lawless, S., Bugajski, D., & Davies, C. (2018). Developing and testing the diagnostic accuracy of a brief nursing dysphagia screen for pneumonia inpatients. *American Journal of Speech-Language Pathology* (In Press).

Hahn, J., Byrd, R., Lengerich, A., Hench, J., Ford, C., Byrd, S., & Stoltz, R. (2015). Neonatal abstinence syndrome: The experience of infant massage. *Creative Nursing, 22*(1), 45–50. doi:10.1891/1078-4535.22.1.45

Honaker, J., Brockopp, D., & Moe, K. (2014). Development and psychometric testing of the Honaker suspected deep tissue injury severity scale. *Journal of Wound, Ostomy and Continence Nursing, 41*(3), 238–241. doi:10.1097/won.0000000000000024

Kjelland, K., Corley, D., Slusher, I., Moe, K., & Brockopp, D. (2018). The Best for Baby Card: An evaluation of factors that influence women's decisions to breastfeed. *Newborn & Infant Nursing Reviews, 14*(1), 23–27. doi:10.1053/j.nainr.2013.12.007

Lengerich, A., Bugajski, A., Marchese, M., Hall, B., Yackzan, S., Davies, C., & Brockopp, D. (2017). The Baptist Health Nurse Retention Questionnaire: A methodological study, part 1. *JONA, 47*(5), 289–293. doi:10.1097/NNA.0000000000000480

Lengerich, A., Brockopp, D., Yackzan, S., Abner, J., Schreiber, J., Hatch, J., . . . , Moe, K. (2018).Women's psychological well-being pre and post-diagnosis of breast cancer: A prospective cohort study. Manuscript submitted for publication.

Lewis, D. A., Sanders, L. P., & Brockopp, D. Y. (2011). The effect of three nursing interventions on thermoregulation in low birth weight infants. *Neonatal Network, 30*(3), 160–164. doi:10.1891 /07300832.30.3.160

Melton, L., Lengerich, A., Collins, M., McKeehan, R., Dunn, D., Griggs, P., . . . , Bugajski, A. (2017). Evaluation of huddles: A multisite study. *Health Care Management (Frederick), 36*(3), 282–287. doi:10.1097/hcm.0000000000000171

Moynahan, S., Swigert, N., Steele, C., & Lengerich, A. (2018). Development of the Baptist Health dysphagia screen for patients postextubation. Manuscript submitted for publication.

Melton, L., Lengerich, A., Collins, M., McKeehan, R., Dunn, D., Griggs, P., Davies, T., Johnson, B., & Bugajski, D. (2017). Evaluation of huddles: A multisite study. *The Health Care Manager, 36*(3), 282–287. doi: 10.1097/HCM.0000000000000171

Norman, D. L., & Streiner, N. (2010). *Health measurement scales: A practical guide to their development and use.* New York, NY: Oxford Press.

Nunnally, J. C. *Psychometric theory* (2nd ed.). New York, NY: McGraw-Hill Book Company.

Pallant, J. (2007). SPSS survival manual (3rd ed.). New York, NY: Open University Press.

Park, M., Kyung, J., Jang, S., & Lee, J. (2017). Evaluating test-retest reliability in patient-reported outcome measures for older people: A systematic review. *International Journal of Nursing Studies, 79,* 58–69.

Paiva, C., Barroso, E., Carnesca, E., Souza, C., Santos, F., Lopez, R., & Paiva, S. (2017). A critical analysis of test-retest reliability in instrument validation studies of cancer patients under palliative care: A systematic review. *BMC: Medical Research Methodology, (14)8.* doi:10.1186/1471-2288-14-8

Polit, D. F., & Beck, C. T. (2017). *Nursing research: Generating and assessing evidence for nursing practice.* Philadelphia, PA: Wolters Kluwer.

Ryff, C. D., & Singer, B. (1998). The contours of positive human health. *Psychological Inquiry, 9*(1), 1.

Stoltz, R., Byrd, R., Hench, A. J., Slone, T., Brockopp, D., & Moe, K. (2014). Does the type of sleep surface influence infant wellbeing in the NICU? *American Journal of Maternal Child Nursing, 39*(6), 363–368. doi:10.1097/nmc.0000000000000078

Thompson, M., Moe, K., & Lewis, C. P. (2014). The effects of music on diminishing anxiety among preoperative patients. *Journal of Radiology Nursing, 33*(4), 199–202. doi:10.1016/j.jradnu.2014.10.005

Waltz, C. F., Strickland, O. L., & Lentz, E. R. (2010). *Measurement in nursing and health research* (4th ed.). New York, NY: Springer Publishing.

Yackzan, S. (2017). Factors influencing preference for surgical choice among women with breast cancer. (Unpublished Dissertation)

Yurdugul, H. (2008). Minimum sample size for Cronbach's coefficient alpha: A Monte-Carlo study. *H.U. Journal of Education, 35,* 397–405.

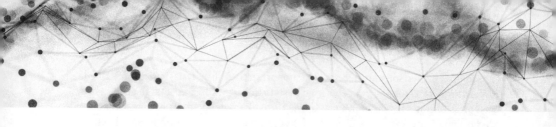

CHAPTER 6

Statistical Analysis: Answering Questions

"The choice of the appropriate statistical method for analyzing data is a crucial factor in the eventual worth of the research project."

— **Brockopp & Hastings-Tolsma**, 2003

▶ Introduction

Statistics is a form of mathematics that enables investigators to describe events and/or establish the likelihood that a hypothesized outcome has occurred. Using statistics, data can be organized, summarized, and analyzed. Organizing and summarizing data require investigators to construct databases. In order to analyze data, investigators need to understand the level of measurement of their data, what statistical tests are appropriate given their data, and how to interpret results of analyses.

There are two major categories of statistics: descriptive and inferential. Descriptive statistics are used to describe a phenomenon or group of participants, while inferential statistics are used to extrapolate that phenomenon to a larger population. Analyses of data in a study may be limited to descriptive statistics, or descriptive statistics may be used along with inferential statistics. Descriptive statistics are not based on probability. Means, medians, modes, and/or frequencies may be used to describe variables of interest.

Outcomes of inferential statistics permit investigators to draw inferences from a sample to a larger population. They can take information gained from studying a sample and state how likely that information will apply to the population of interest. The concept of statistical significance conveys the likelihood that the same results will occur by chance rather than the manipulation of a variable.

Within inferential statistics there are two groups of tests: parametric and nonparametric. Parametric tests have a prescribed set of assumptions underlying their use, while nonparametric tests do not. Nonparametric tests are most useful when data are categorical or ordinal, the distribution is clearly nonnormal, or the sample is small.

In this chapter, software necessary to support statistical analysis is briefly described, explanations of terms and concepts used in statistics are addressed, and the two major categories of statistics (inferential and descriptive) are detailed. Basic statistical tests are presented and examples from studies conducted in this research-friendly environment (RFE) are included. For investigators interested in advanced statistics, the following texts are recommended: *Discovering Statistics Through SPSS* (Field, 2009), *SPSS Survival Manual* (Pallant, 2010), and *Using Multivariate Statistics* (Tabachnick & Fidell, 2007).

▶ Computer Software

A critical step in the research process, and one of the primary responsibilities of consultants, is to build databases. Once the database is complete, investigators work with a consultant to understand how to input data. Similarly, when data are ready to be analyzed, investigators and consultants work together so that investigators understand the process and the outcome. This RFE has a number of licenses for computer software. Because a limited number of users can have access at a given point in time, access to these licenses can be modified depending on investigators' needs. Access can be assigned to investigators for the duration of their study, and once a study is complete, that license can be assigned to another individual. Each research consultant has ongoing access.

Computer software that is user friendly and readily available is a required resource for the research office. There are numerous statistical software options available on the market that fit these criteria, such as R, SAS, JMP, MatLab, and SPSS. The Statistical Package for the Social Sciences (SPSS; IBM, 2012) is used in this RFE. Investigators are strongly encouraged to enter their data directly into this program because moving data from one program to another, although possible, can be time consuming. How data have been entered into another program is also a consideration in terms of its transferability. If data have been entered into a different program in a manner that makes transfer relatively easy, consultants will transfer those data into SPSS.

At the beginning of this RFE, one SPSS license was available to the one research consultant in the research office. As productivity increased and additional consultants joined the office, additional licenses were purchased. While a few caregivers in the institution prefer other statistical packages, understanding one program well has enabled caregivers and consultants to reduce the amount of time and energy needed for developing databases and analyzing data.

▶ Explanation of Statistical Terms and Concepts

The Hospital-Based Guide to Statistical Analysis (**FIGURE 6-1**) describes the thinking underlying the use of statistics to analyze data. The most frequently used statistical tests in this RFE are included. Each component of the guide will be addressed and examples provided. Guidance in using advanced statistical tests is available in books devoted to statistics (e.g., Tabachnick & Fidell, 2007).

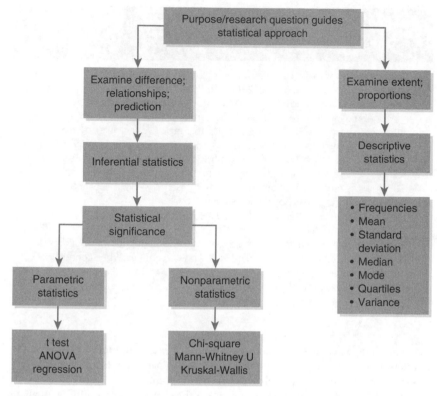

FIGURE 6-1 The Hospital-Based Guide to Statistical Analysis.

Learning statistics is similar to learning a language. There are a number of terms and concepts that are not used in everyday speech, and some words, such as *significance*, have a meaning that differs from usual use. In general usage, significant means important. However, the word *significant*, when used in a statistical context, refers to the likelihood that a result occurred due to the manipulation of an independent variable or the likelihood it occurred by chance. Unfortunately, the concept of probability appears to be difficult for some to understand. The word *proven* is frequently used in discussing research findings when, in actuality, findings only represent the probability of an outcome.

An understanding of the processes and language used in statistics is essential to understanding how variables are measured, how data are analyzed, and how to read statistical results. Some of the terms addressed in this chapter were also described in Chapter 5. They are repeated here because they are important components in the measurement process and equally important in trying to understand statistical analysis.

Variables

Every research question involves variables. For example, in an ongoing study in this RFE, investigators are concerned about occupational safety. They are asking the research question, "What symptoms do medical imaging technologists experience

BOX 6-1 Melanie Thompson, RN: The Effects of Music on Diminishing Anxiety Among Preoperative Patients

In Melanie's study examining the effect of music on anxiety among adult patients prior to surgery (Thompson, Moe, & Lewis, 2014), she reported the difference in the number of participants in each group (music and nonmusic) and assessed the variables of gender, age, and invasiveness of surgery in her sample. With a sample size of 137, she reported that 59 females (80.8%) participated in the music group, while 64 females (75%) were in the no music group. The average age in the music group was 54.64 years, standard deviation (SD) = 12.81; in the nonmusic group, average age was 48.78 years with an SD of 15.13. (The standard deviation represents the average amount values deviate from the mean.) In relation to invasiveness of surgery, 48 participants (40%) had invasive surgery, and 89 had noninvasive surgery (60%).

Melanie used inferential statistics (chi-square, χ^2) to examine differences in gender in both groups. The difference was not significant (χ^2 [1, N=137] = 0.38, p <0.54). This finding suggests that the differences in gender in the music and nonmusic groups likely occurred by chance. For Melanie's study, that finding was positive. When conducting experiments or quasi-experiments, it is important to have membership in different groups as similar as possible.

as the result of exposure to static magnetic fields?" Here, symptoms are the variables of interest. A list of specific symptoms is provided to participants in order to obtain information regarding the prevalence of each symptom.

A variable, from a statistical perspective, is the characteristic, entity, or attribute that has been measured. Examples of variables analyzed in this RFE are satisfaction, comfort, temperature of infants, anxiety, well-being, age, and gender. The number associated with a variable may be used to describe a participant characteristic, such as age or gender. That number may also be used to analyze differences among variables. An example of using variables to describe participants in a study is presented in **BOX 6-1**.

Independent and Dependent Variables

The terms *independent variable* and *dependent variable* are used to describe two important components of the research process. The independent variable may refer to an intervention, such as music, as in the study described in Box 5-1. It may also refer to a construct, such as self-confidence. In the research question, "What is the effect of confidence on nurses' competence to care for patients?," confidence would be the independent variable. The independent variable is hypothesized to affect the dependent variable.

The dependent variable is the variable of interest to the investigator. It is "acted on" by the independent variable. In the study conducted in this RFE to examine the effects of three interventions on neonates' temperatures (Lewis, Sanders, & Brockopp, 2011), temperature is the dependent variable, and the three interventions were the independent variables. The investigator was interested in problems related to thermoregulation among these babies. She looked at differences in temperature (dependent variable) following three interventions designed to improve thermoregulation. Another example of independent and dependent variables is provided in **BOX 6-2**.

BOX 6-2 Holly Weyl, RN, BSN, OCN: Understanding Colorectal Screening Behaviors and Factors Associated with Screening in a Community Hospital Setting

Holly conducted a quasi-experiment to examine the effects of educational materials on colorectal screening (Weyl et al., 2015). Participants (N=167) received educational materials regarding the importance of screening in the mail. Following receipt of the materials, they were called on the telephone by the investigator. Participants responded to a structured telephone interview. Data on reasons for not being screened, as well as whether or not their healthcare providers had discussed the importance of screening, were collected. The independent variable was the educational materials provided to participants. Dependent variables included reasons for not being screened and whether or not healthcare providers discussed the importance of screening with them.

Levels of Measurement

As caregivers and research consultants work together to discuss how data will be analyzed, they identify the level of available data. Data can be characterized as nominal, ordinal, interval, and ratio. Nominal data may also be referred to as categorical. For example, sex is an example of nominal data, as it represents two distinct categories. Variables may also be modified to provide nominal data rather than continuous data. For example, in some studies, investigators may collapse data collected on age into two groups (e.g., 49 years or younger and 50 years or older).

Ordinal data differ from nominal data in that the categories of information are rank ordered along a specific dimension. The distance among categories is unknown. An example of ordinal data in a hospital study might be patient responses to functional ability. Participants might respond to an item about mobility with one of the following options: (1) able to walk without assistance, (2) able to walk with a little assistance, (3) able to walk with a lot of assistance. The distance between each assessment of walking (i.e., the difference between "a little" and "a lot") may be quite different. The important point is that this distance cannot be considered equal.

Interval data are also rank ordered. The assumption, however, is that the space between each value is equal. In addition, interval data are not required to reflect a variable that has an absolute zero (i.e., the absence of the variable). Temperature is an example of interval data. The difference between 75 and 80 degrees is the same as the difference between 25 and 30 degrees. Furthermore, temperature has no natural zero point because 0 degrees does not mean an absence of temperature.

Ratio is another category of measurement. Ratio data are interval data that have an absolute zero point. For example, when measuring distance, a distance of 0 means that no distance was traveled.

Identification of the level of measurement of a variable is required before decisions can be made regarding analysis of data. Research consultants in this RFE recommend that statistical analysis of data is discussed and decisions made at the outset of the caregiver's study. The goal of consultants is to have caregivers, from the beginning, understand their studies from research question to possible results. Understanding measurement levels and statistical tests from the beginning of their study enables caregivers to make appropriate decisions about the data they will collect. This process

> **BOX 6-3** Regina Stoltz, RN, ARNP, PNP-BC: Does the Type of Sleep Surface Influence Infant Well-Being in the NICU?
>
> Regina assessed the effect of sleep surface on infant well-being in the NICU (Stoltz et al., 2014). She collected data on sex, birthweight, and parents' perception of infants' comfort level. Sex was indicated as either male or female, which represents nominal data. Birthweight is interval data, in that the difference between each gram of weight is the same. Parents rated their infant's well-being as irritable/restless (score of 1), somewhat comfortable (score of 2), and very comfortable (score of 3); responses to these items are categorized as ordinal data. Choice of statistical analysis was based on each type of data collected. Differences in sex were analyzed using chi-square (χ^2), while birthweight differences were analyzed using a t test.

also appears to diminish some of the mystery associated with statistics. An example of a study that included ordinal and interval data is provided in **BOX 6-3**.

Statistical Significance

> Statistical
> significance

Traditionally, statistical significance refers to the likelihood that results of a study occurred by chance rather than the influence of an independent variable on one or more dependent variables. Statistical significance has been set as equal to or less than a cutoff score of 0.05. This number is referred to as an alpha level. Results of data analyses report findings in terms of significance as a p value. For example, $p < 0.01$ means that the result of the statistical test suggests that this finding would be due to chance 1 time out of 100, or this finding could be interpreted as the result occurring 99 times out of 100.

The independent variable in the study in Box 6-3 is an experimental sleep surface. In this study, if the author had hypothesized that infant weight would increase due to the experimental sleep surface, and her analysis revealed a probability level of less than 0.05 ($p < 0.05$) she could state that the weight gain was statistically significant. A significant finding ($p < 0.05$) related to weight gain would tell her that only 5 times out of 100 would her finding be due to chance and not the experimental mattress. Caregivers in this RFE often confuse the idea of significance with clinical importance. While establishing how likely an independent variable (sleep surface) is to impact a dependent variable (weight gain) is important when conducting research, that finding should not be translated as clinically meaningful (Polit & Beck, 2016). The difference in weight needs to be examined in terms of clinical importance. An example of a calculation of statistical significance is provided in **BOX 6-4**.

Means, Medians, and Modes

Means, medians, and modes are calculations that are frequently used when analyzing data. The goal of these calculations is to describe how typical a given number is in a

BOX 6-4 Preston Lewis, RN, DNP, MSN, CCRN: Overcoming Barriers to Effective Pain Management: The Use of Professionally Directed Small Group Discussions

In an effort to improve the management of pain on critical care units, Preston designed a study to evaluate the use of professionally directed small group discussions (independent variable) on barriers (dependent variables) to effective pain management (Lewis, Corley, Lake, Brockopp, & Moe, 2015). Knowledge of pain management was one of the dependent variables he assessed. Results of a t test showed a significant difference in knowledge, in a positive direction, following group discussions within 3 months post intervention. At an alpha level of 0.001 (p <0.001), this finding suggests that this change in knowledge would occur by chance only 1 time out of 1,000.

data set. Given that the most typical number is more likely to occur in the center of a distribution of numbers as opposed to the extreme, means, medians, and modes are termed measures of central tendency. A mean is the average of a group of scores. It is calculated by adding a group of scores and dividing by the number of cases. For example, if an investigator wants to find the mean of 10 scores on a questionnaire, with scores ranging from 1 to 25, those scores would be added and divided by 10. Of the three indexes, the mean is most often used in research. It is the most stable of the three indexes of "typicalness." When means, medians, and modes are calculated in a given population, the mean varies the least.

Medians are the middle score in a set of ordered observations. When there is an even number of scores, the median is the average of the two scores that fall on either side of what would be the middle score. The mode is the most frequently occurring score in a data set.

▶ Type I and Type II Errors

There are two types of hypotheses: the research hypothesis and the null hypothesis. The research hypothesis reflects the outcome desired by the investigator, and the null hypothesis states that there will be no difference. For example, the investigator in the pain study described in Box 6-4 hypothesized that group discussions would improve nurses' knowledge regarding pain management (research hypothesis). As such, the null hypothesis for the pain study would state that there would be no difference in knowledge of pain management scores following group discussions.

Investigators use a variety of statistical tests with the goal of rejecting the null hypothesis. Because investigators cannot know with certainty whether or not the null hypothesis is true based on data from a sample, a risk of error is always present. There are two types of possible errors. A type I error occurs when the investigator concludes that a difference or relationship among variables exists when it does not (a false positive). A type II error occurs when the investigator concludes that a difference or relationship does not exist when it does (a false negative). Statistical analysis in many instances is a response to hypothesis testing. The concepts of type I and type II errors affirm the idea that statistical analysis does not provide proof—there is always a possibility that findings are due to chance.

Confidence Intervals

Taking information gained from a sample and accurately translating that information to the larger population is a basic goal of statistical analysis. In order to estimate a parameter (e.g., mean, proportion) from a sample that will reflect the variable of interest in the population, various statistical tests are performed. For example, the mean score on the pain knowledge questionnaire, from Box 6-4, was calculated. That mean was considered to be representative of scores that could apply to the larger population of nurses. Identifying a mean score given a particular level of probability is called point estimation. Conclusions are drawn from one mean value.

Interval estimation is another approach to identifying a parameter that can reflect the means of many samples within a population. For example, the mean of nurses' competency scores on pain control may be 14 using a 25-item measure. If that assessment were conducted on several other samples of nurses, discovering that exact mean for each sample is unlikely. The range of means allows for the possibility that the mean is within a specified set of values. Using interval estimation, investigators are able to construct a confidence interval around a sample mean. This confidence interval is usually established using an alpha level (probability) of 0.05 or 0.99 (Polit & Beck, 2016). An example of establishing a confidence interval is provided in **BOX 6-5**.

Power Analysis

The size of a sample can influence the outcome of statistical analyses. Analyzing data from a sample that is too small can diminish the probability of reaching statistical significance and lead to type I (false positive) and type II (false negative) errors. In order to calculate a sample size (power analysis) that has a strong probability of reaching significance, the appropriate statistical test must be selected. The choice of test is guided by the research question and the variables under consideration. The goal of investigators may be to examine relationships, test differences, or predict specific outcomes. Depending on the goal of the researcher, the statistical test can be identified.

 BOX 6-5 Claire Davies, PT, PhD: Test–Retest and Internal Consistency of the Disability of Arm, Shoulder and Hand (DASH) Outcome Measure in Assessing Functional Status Among Breast Cancer Survivors with Lymphedema

Claire tested the use of Astym therapy, a treatment approach to soft-tissue injuries, among women following mastectomy (Davies, Brockopp, & Moe, 2015). She was interested in the treatment's effect on functioning. She used the Disability of Arm, Shoulder and Hand (DASH) questionnaire, a 30-item, self-report measure, that includes items related to social, physical, and psychological functioning. Participants responded to the questionnaire before and after the Astym therapy treatment. She analyzed her data using a t test and found a significant (p <0.01) positive difference in functioning following the Astym therapy treatment. She calculated a confidence interval of 3.95–15.72. This finding suggests that the mean score of several samples would likely fall within that interval.

BOX 6-6 Jeremy Honaker, RN, BSN, CWOCN: The Effect of Adjunctive Noncontact Low-Frequency Ultrasound on Deep-Tissue Pressure Injury

Jeremy conducted a study to examine the effect of low-frequency ultrasound on healing of suspected deep-tissue injury (SDTI) (Honaker, Forston, Davis, Wiesner, & Morgan, 2012). Jeremy and his team conducted a retrospective chart review to assess treatment effectiveness as measured by the Honaker Suspected Deep Tissue injury Scale and final pressure ulcer stage. They collected data from the charts on patients with SDTI who experienced the treatment and those who did not and used t tests to assess differences between groups. In order to discover how many patients were needed in each group to have an 85% chance of achieving significance, they conducted a power analysis. With p=0.05 and a moderate effect size, they found they needed 63 patients in each group.

In addition to the statistical test (t test, chi-square, etc.) that will be used to analyze the data, a power analysis calculation requires investigators to select an alpha level (e.g., $p < 0.05$, <0.01), an effect size (to what degree will the independent variable influence the dependent variable), and the power desired. An investigator may want an 80% chance of achieving significance, determined as an 85% chance or higher. As the power desired increases, so must the sample size. Inserting these data into a computer program will provide the sample size required. G power is the most commonly used statistical package for conducting power analyses. A power analysis was calculated in the study described in **BOX 6-6**.

Statistical Terms and Concepts: Summary

Knowledge of the terms and concepts described above is helpful if caregivers want to understand how to analyze their data and publish their results. In this RFE, new investigators learn these terms and concepts as they design and conduct their studies.

▶ Inferential Statistics

Inferential statistics

Investigators who use inferential statistics want to make an inference from the sample studied to the population of interest. For example, the investigator who examined the association between screening for colorectal cancer and having access to a healthcare provider who discussed the importance of screening (Weyl et al., 2015) was able to infer that this kind of access does influence screening in a positive direction. Statistical significance was found and the difference between the two groups—screened and not screened—was clinically meaningful. In this case, a nonparametric statistical test was calculated. Differences in nonparametric and parametric tests are described below. Examples of basic statistical tests frequently used in this RFE are also included.

Parametric and Nonparametric Statistics

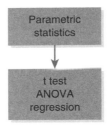

Within statistics there are two broad classifications of statistical tests: parametric and nonparametric. Parametric tests are more powerful than nonparametric tests. They are based on a number of assumptions and are usually preferred. A conservative approach to statistical analysis insists that if parametric tests are used, the assumptions must be met. There is evidence, however, to suggest that if a sample size is sufficiently large, violation of these assumptions does not affect outcomes (Polit & Beck, 2016).

Normal distribution of the variables under consideration is one of the assumptions underlying the use of parametric tests. However, if a sample size is 50 or greater, even though the variables of interest are not normally distributed, parametric tests may be used. Central limit theorem states that when samples are large, the theoretical distribution of means tends to be normally distributed (Polit & Beck, 2016).

Assumptions of Parametric Statistics

Normal Distribution. The availability of normally distributed data is the most emphasized assumption of parametric tests. Normal distribution can be likened to a bell curve where the peak is exactly halfway between each tail. The issue of normality is addressed differently depending on the type of statistical test. Tests used in this RFE assume that the sampling distribution (the distribution of data that were collected during the study) is normal. The role of normality using more complex and advanced statistics can be found in Tabachnick and Fidell (2007).

Homogeneity of Variance. Homogeneity of variance is another assumption underlying parametric statistics. This assumption means that data from multiple groups have the same variance. Using the development of the high-risk falls assessment (Corley et al., 2014) as an example, 241,599 assessments of falls were collected at four different hospitals. The mean age of patients was the same at three hospitals (M= 65 years). Even though the means were the same, the variation in ages in each sample was different. That variation refers to homogeneity of variance. An index of variability can be calculated to describe the degree to which scores, or in this case age, vary in a particular distribution (Polit & Beck, 2016).

Interval or Ratio Data. Parametric tests are conducted on data that are continuous, such as interval or ratio. As mentioned previously, there is an assumption if using interval data that the space between each number of a scale is the same. Parametric tests cannot be conducted using data that are nominal or ordinal. There are nonparametric tests that can be used with these two types of data.

Independence. The assumption of independence means that the data from one participant are independent (not related) to the data from another participant. However, there are examples of statistical tests (e.g., repeated measures analysis of variance) where it is expected that this assumption is violated.

Parametric Statistical Tests: Relationship

Correlation in statistics refers to the relationship, sometimes known as an association, between two or more variables. A coefficient can be calculated that will describe the extent of the relationship and whether it is in a positive or negative direction. It is important to note that caution should be used interpreting correlation coefficients. Relationships between variables do not translate to causation.

If nurses' scores on a questionnaire measuring their knowledge of pain are analyzed to detect a relationship with years of nursing experience, there may be a positive relationship. However, that does not suggest that years of experience are the cause of increased knowledge regarding pain management. A correlation coefficient can range from −1 to +1, with a coefficient of −1 indicating a perfect negative relationship, +1 indicating a perfect positive relationship, and 0 indicating no relationship. The calculation of r^2 describes the percentage of variance in one variable that can be explained by another variable. A correlation coefficient is calculated in the study described in **BOX 6-7**.

Correlational Statistical Tests

Based on level of data collected, there are different statistical tests used to establish relationships among variables. Pearson Product Moment, point-biserial, and intraclass correlation are three frequently used in this RFE and described below. The Pearson Product Moment correlation (Pearson r) is the most commonly used test when describing relationships among variables. In order to calculate this coefficient, data must be interval or ratio. Two sets of numerical data are required. Attempting to identify a relationship between age (numerical) and weight (numerical) is an example of data that would be appropriate for calculating a Pearson r. If there was a negative relationship between those two variables, it could be written $r = -0.45$. A positive

 BOX 6-7 Jeremy Honaker, RN, BSN, CWOCN: Development and Psychometric Testing of the Honaker Suspected Deep Tissue Injury (SDTI) Severity Scale

Jeremy conducted a study to test an instrument he designed to detect suspected deep-tissue injuries (SDTIs) (Honaker, Brockopp, & Moe, 2014). As part of the development process, he asked 21 healthcare providers (6 physical therapists and 15 nurses) to examine photographs of 3 patients with SDTIs upon initial assessment and at discharge. They were instructed to rate these photographs using the scale Jeremy constructed. They provided a total of 126 ratings. A correlation coefficient was calculated ($r = 0.99$, $p < 0.001$). This finding suggests an outstanding relationship among healthcare professionals' ratings of the instrument.

BOX 6-8 Claire Davies, PT, PhD: Internal Consistency of the Disability of Arm, Shoulder and Hand (DASH) Outcome Measure in Assessing Functional Status Among Breast Cancer Survivors

Claire tested the reliability (consistency over time) of the Disability of Arm, Shoulder and Hand (DASH) outcome measure among breast cancer survivors (Davies, Brockopp, & Moe, 2015). This instrument had not been tested on this particular population. Participants completed the DASH, in person, at their initial physical therapy visit and a second time 2 to 3 hours later on the telephone. The goal was to see how closely participants' first scores on the DASH matched their scores when they responded to the measure a second time. She calculated an Intraclass Correlation Coefficient (ICC) (0.97) and a confidence interval (0.93–0.99). Her result showed an excellent relationship of scores over time.

relationship would be stated as $r = 0.45$). Significance, the likelihood of this finding occurring again given the same situation, is also reported ($p < 0.05$).

A point-biserial correlation coefficient is a special type of the Pearson Product Moment correlation. It can be calculated between a dichotomous variable and a continuous variable. For example, a caregiver who wants to examine the relationship between membership in a group and a dependent variable could use this test. A study designed to assess the relationship between nurse education (ADN and BSN) and scores on a competency exam could calculate a point biserial correlation coefficient. An intraclass correlation coefficient (ICC) compares the variability of scores within a group to the variability of scores across groups. The ICC is the preferred statistical test when assessing the reliability (test–retest) of a measure (see **BOX 6-8**).

Parametric Statistical Tests: Testing Mean Differences Between Two Groups

Caregivers may want to examine differences in a dependent variable following an intervention or differences among existing groups. Often in this RFE, differences in dependent variables between two groups are analyzed. Examples include differences in anxiety between a group of patients who experienced music prior to surgery and a group who did not, temperatures among infants exposed to three interventions related to thermoregulation and those who were not, and nurses' knowledge and assessment of patients' pain who experienced an intervention and those who did not.

Statistical Tests for Difference

T tests are appropriate statistical tests when examining a difference between two groups. These tests evaluate the difference between two means. Independent t tests are used when the groups differ. In each of the above examples, participants in one group were not the same individuals as in the second group—that is, presurgery patients who listened to music were different from patients who did not listen to music.

Dependent t tests are calculated when the same individuals are assessed on two different occasions. For example, in a study to overcome barriers to effective pain management (Lewis et al., 2015), a group of nurses (N=32) completed a questionnaire before an intervention and after the intervention. Because the same individuals were involved, a dependent t test was calculated.

There are advantages in designing a study that examines responses of the same participants on two different occasions. Characteristics such as personality, health, income, and many more can influence a participant's response to an assessment. If the same individuals are assessed on two occasions, there is less fluctuation in the sample based on issues not related to the study.

At a practical level, however, collecting useable data from the same participants on two occasions can be challenging. In order to calculate a dependent t test, an identifier needs to be attached to each participant's response. Data must be matched to each participant on time one and time two. Personal identification is not supported by institutional research boards, and other kinds of identifiers, such as "mother's birthday" may not be reported the same the second time participants respond to the questionnaire. In this RFE, approximately 15% of data using an identifier cannot be used because of mismatches. An example of findings analyzed using a t test is described in **BOX 6-9**.

In the example described above, the t value (1.89) is the outcome of a mathematical calculation that enables the discovery of a probability value (p <0.02). The numerical value 58 reflects the degrees of freedom—that is, the number of values in the statistical calculation that are free to vary. The most important value in the reporting of the t test is the p value. In this case, a p value of 0.02 (<0.05) established that the result is significant. Computer software allows the investigator to enter appropriate data, identify the desired statistical test, and quickly receive the values described above.

A problem can occur when investigators use t tests to analyze the differences between means of a number of variables in the same data set. As the number of t tests calculated increases, the possibility of incurring a type I error (the investigator concludes that a difference or relationship among variables exists when it does not) also increases.

There are two options when this situation occurs. A Bonferroni correction can be calculated. This formula sets a probability value that will account for the number

 BOX 6-9 Judith Schreiber, RN, MSN, PhD: Improving Knowledge, Assessment, and Attitudes Related to Pain Management

Judith designed a study to improve nurses' knowledge, assessment, and attitudes related to pain management (Schreiber et al., 2014). As a component of the study, patients (N=60) recorded numerical assessments of their pain (0 [no pain] to 10 [extreme pain]) in a pain diary. One of the questions addressed in this study was "What is the difference in agreement between nurses' assessment of patients' pain, reflected in their charting, and patients' assessment of their pain in their diaries?" Thirty nurses participated in an educational intervention, and 30 did not. Mean scores for differences in assessments were calculated. An independent t test (t [58] = 1.89, p <0.02) followed. Results suggest that nurses who obtain additional information regarding pain control assess pain more closely to patients' assessments than nurses who do not receive additional information. The difference in pain assessments was considered meaningful.

BOX 6-10   Krista Moe, PhD: Major Predictors of Inpatient Falls: A Multisite Study

Krista conducted a secondary data analysis on a large data set (N=281,865) collected during the development of a high-risk falls assessment (Moe, Brockopp, McCowan, Merritt, & Hall, 2015). She wanted to identify key factors predictive of inpatient falls. Her analysis included data related to seven variables: age, gender, confusion, toileting issues, mobility, sedation, and nurse's clinical judgment regarding fall risk. Because seven tests would be used, thereby increasing the chances of type I errors, she conducted a Bonferroni correction. As a result, her alpha level was reduced to 0.01. In order to reach significance, the probability of results being due to chance would be raised from the standard 5 times out of 10 to 1 time out of 100.

of statistical tests calculated in one data set. As the number of calculations increases, the probability level decreases. A second option is to use a statistical test (analysis of variance [ANOVA]) that is effective when assessing difference and does not result in a possible increase in type I errors. An example of using a Bonferroni correction is described in **BOX 6-10**.

Statistical Tests: Testing Mean Differences Among More Than Two Groups

Analysis of variance (ANOVA) is a statistical test that enables an investigator to compare mean differences among two or more groups on a particular measure. The one-way ANOVA is the most frequently used statistical test to accomplish this goal. Using one-way ANOVA, the independent variable is nominal and has two or more levels. For example, sex has two levels: male and female. Dependent variables are continuous (interval or ratio). One-way ANOVA is used when there is only one dependent variable (the outcome variable).

Two-way ANOVA indicates that there are two independent variables. This test examines the variability of means between independent groups and contrasts that variability with the variance within groups. An independent group is one in which participants in the groups studied are not the same (i.e., participants in one group are not matched with participants in another group).

If results show that the variance within groups and between groups is similar or the same, no difference is found. An F ratio provides a numerical value that reflects the between-group variability over the within-group variability. This value needs to be greater than 1 if a difference in variables studied exists. The F ratio enables the identification of the probability level (p).

Two terms are used when discussing ANOVA: main effect and interaction. The main effect refers to the effect of one independent variable on a dependent variable. Interaction describes the effect of two or more independent variables (acting together) on a dependent variable. For example, three groups of nurses are formed—one group has 2 years of nursing experience, one group has 5 years of experience, and the third group has 20. An educational workshop is designed to motivate these nurses to remain in a given acute care setting. The first group has the experience; the second group has the experience plus receives a salary bonus, and the third does not receive either intervention. Intent to stay is measured in all groups.

The null hypothesis would be that all "intent to stay" scores are the same. The results of one-way ANOVA will provide information related to whether there is a difference among groups. In order to discover where the difference exists, another test, termed *post hoc*, is required. The Sheffe test and Fisher's least significant difference test are two post hoc tests that may be used. **BOX 6-11** describes the use of ANOVA in a nurse retention study.

Statistical tests described thus far are applied to data that are collected at two points in time. When making particular changes in practice, however, caregivers may want to assess a variable on multiple occasions. For example, changes made related to discharge planning may be sustained for 1 month or 2, but do they still exist 6 months later? In addition to caregivers' concerns, criteria for Magnet designation require that data be collected following an intervention on three occasions post intervention (ANCC, 2013).

A repeated measures ANOVA (RMANOVA) is the most appropriate statistical test to use when means are calculated for the same participants at three or more points in time. A one-way repeated measures ANOVA is an extension of a dependent t test, while the simple one-way ANOVA is an extension of an independent t test. Participants in the RMANOVA are related, while participants in one-way ANOVA are independent of one another. Interpretation of results is the same for RMANOVA as one-way ANOVA. An example of RM ANOVA is presented in **BOX 6-12**.

Analysis of covariance (ANCOVA) is used when investigators want to understand the difference among two or more groups while controlling for specific variables. For example, if a team of caregivers wanted to study mobility following surgery, at 3 months, 6 months, and 12 months, and wanted to control for the age of patients, they could use ANCOVA to analyze their data.

Parametric Statistical Tests: Prediction

Regression analysis is a statistical approach to predicting change in a dependent variable (e.g., length of stay on a particular hospital unit) on the basis of a change in one or more independent variables (e.g., increasing number of discharge planners and adoption of new medications). There are two categories of regression analyses: simple linear and multiple. Both categories are based on correlational techniques.

BOX 6-12 Regina Stoltz, RN, ARNP, PNP-BC: Staff Nurse Perceptions of Open Pod and Single-Family-Room NICU Designs on Work Environment and Patient Care

Before a planned environmental change occurred in the neonatal intensive care unit (NICU), the director of the NICU designed a study to assess nurses' perceptions regarding two different workspaces: open pod and single-family rooms (Winner-Stoltz et al., 2018). Originally, nurses were taking care of patients in an open pod arrangement. The move would require them to work in single-family rooms. Questionnaires designed to evaluate nurses' perceptions of their workspace were completed 6 months prior to the move and at 3, 9, and 15 months post move. The questionnaire contained eight domains related to nurses' perceptions. Significant differences were found in six of the eight domains. For example, a significant difference regarding environmental quality and control of primary workspace was found ($F[3, 78] = 26.912$, $p < 0.001$). The finding favored the single-family-room workspace. The greatest change in perception occurred at the first time point following the move.

Simple linear regression involves using one independent variable (e.g., patients' functional status post surgery) to predict a dependent variable (e.g., length of hospital stay). If the relationship between these two variables is linear and perfect, knowledge of one variable enables the prediction of the other. While a correlation coefficient (Pearson's r) could be calculated to provide information regarding the extent of the relationship, linear regression enables prediction.

Rarely is the relationship between two variables perfect. If it were perfect, a straight line could represent the values analyzed. Regression techniques identify the straight line that runs through the data points with the best possible fit. A regression equation is a formula used to define the best-fitting straight line that characterizes the relationship between the two variables. The result is reported as R^2.

Multiple regression involves multiple independent variables, often referred to as predictor variables. For example, if investigators were interested in the relationship between mobility and length of stay following surgery, a correlation coefficient could be calculated. If they wanted to predict the influence of mobility, age, and weight on length of stay, they could use multiple regression.

Unfortunately, when predictor variables are highly correlated with each other, predictive value diminishes. For example, age and mobility could be highly correlated. A strong correlation among predictor variables is termed *multicollinearity*. Calculations can detect the degree of multicollinearity in a set of variables. R^2 is calculated for predictor variables.

While linear and multiple regression require data that are interval or ratio level, logistic regression is used to analyze relationships between a categorical variable (e.g., 30-day readmission to hospital) and two or more dependent variables (e.g., age and income). This test is similar to multiple regression in that it is used to analyze the relationship among independent variables and one dependent variable.

Odds ratios are frequently calculated to express the relative risk of an occurrence. The odds ratio is defined as the likelihood of an occurrence compared to the likelihood of nonoccurrence. For example, if multimodal pain management is used with one group of patients and traditional pain management is used with a similar group of patients, the odds ratio would reflect how likely pain scores in the experimental group would be acceptable compared to the likelihood that pain scores would be acceptable in the control group. Values of the odds ratio less than 1 are considered decreased odds, and greater than 1 are increased odds. A value equal to 1 means the odds of pain scores being acceptable (the outcome of interest) are no greater than chance. A study designed to examine predictors of inpatient falls using logistic regression is described in **BOX 6-13**.

Nonparametric Statistical Tests: Association

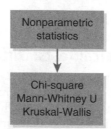

Chi-square (χ^2) is the nonparametric test used most frequently by researchers. Chi-square analyses are used to make inferences about the existence of a relationship between two categorical variables. Data collected to understand the difference between the number of male nurses on the night shift as opposed to the day shift could be analyzed using chi-square. Sex (male or female) and shift (night shift, day shift) are the two categorical variables. The contingency table is an example of data organized for chi-square analysis (**TABLE 6-1**).

From examining the contingency table, there are fewer females working the night shift compared to the day shift and more males working the night shift than the day shift. Calculation of a Pearson's chi-square test provides information regarding whether or not the differences seen in the table are significant. For this example, the chi-square statistic (χ^2) is 4.336, and the p value is 0.03. There is a significant difference between men working the night shift and day shift. Results from the study described in **BOX 6-14** were calculated using chi-square (χ^2).

TABLE 6-1 Contingency Table for Chi-Square (χ^2) Analysis

	Day Shift	Night Shift	Total
Male	5	13	18
Female	45	37	82
Total	50	50	100

BOX 6-14 Kim Kjelland, RN, MSN, PNP-BC: The Best for Baby Card—An Evaluation of Factors That Influence Women's Decisions to Breastfeed

Kim investigated the effect of a small laminated card (Best for Baby Card) on women's decisions to breastfeed. She also examined factors that influence this decision (Kjelland, Corley, Slusher, Moe, & Brockopp, 2014). Using a chi-square test for independence, her team did not find a significant difference in decisions to breastfeed (yes, no) and receipt of the card (yes, no) (χ^2 [1, N=20] =0.30, p = 0.58). Significant associations were found for response to a number of factors related to the decision to breastfeed. For example, women who breastfed made the decision to breastfeed prior to pregnancy (χ^2 [1, N=120] = 66.56, p <0.001), had support from their partner to breastfeed (χ^2 [1, N=112] = 17.93, p <0.001), and breastfed the infant within 1 hour of birth (χ^2 [1, N=120] = 30.59, p <0.001).

Nonparametric Statistical Tests: Difference

The Mann-Whitney U test or Wilcoxon rank sum test is a nonparametric test used to compare differences between two independent groups when the dependent variable is either ordinal or continuous but not normally distributed. It is similar to an independent t test in that participants are not the same in both groups.

For example, a researcher is interested in examining the differences in mean satisfaction scores between male and female patients on a given nursing unit. Following data collection, the researcher discovers that responses from male patients are not normally distributed. Scores related to female patients' responses are normally distributed. Normal distribution resembles a bell curve (see **FIGURE 6-2**).

Initially, the researcher may have intended to analyze the scores between the two groups by conducting an independent t test. On discovering that one group's data are skewed, calculating a Mann-Whitney U would be an appropriate choice (**FIGURE 6-3**).

When the analyses are conducted, the output will provide the researcher with four test statistics: Mann-Whitney U, Wilcoxon W, z score, and significance level (p value). The Mann-Whitney U and Wilcoxon statistics are derived by ranking the scores in each group from lowest to highest and then adding the ranks (see **TABLE 6-2**). The z score is a standardized score that enables calculations leading to a decision regarding significance (probability that the difference did not occur by chance, identified by p <0.05). This test can be used with small sample sizes with good results.

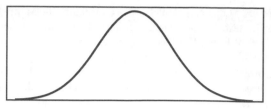

FIGURE 6-2 Female patients' distribution of satisfaction scores.

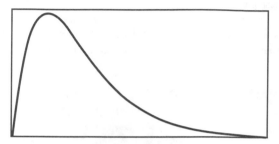

FIGURE 6-3 Men's distribution of satisfaction scores. This is a skewed distribution and is not normal.

TABLE 6-2 Example of How to Rank Data

Total Satisfaction Score	10 11 **12 12** 14 15 16 22 24 26 27 **32 32 32 32** 33 34 35 36 37
Potential Rank	1 2 **3 4** 5 6 7 8 9 10 11 **12 13 14 15** 16 17 18 19 20
Actual Rank	1 2 **3.5** 5 6 7 8 9 10 11 **13.5** 16 17 18 19 20
Group (male or female)	M F M M M F F M M M F M M M F F F F F F

In order to use this statistical test, data are rank ordered. Scores in each group are ranked from lowest to highest. If there are multiples of raw data scores (see bolded scores), rankings are averaged (i.e., [3 + 4]/2 = 3.5). Rankings are summed and averaged.

The Wilcoxon signed rank test is the nonparametric equivalent of an independent t test. This test is used to examine how participants change over time. Instead of two groups, there are two time points. Similar to the example in Table 6-2, raw data are ranked. Ranking is completed by taking the difference between Time 2 and Time 1. Differences in the median values between participants in the control group as opposed to the experimental group are calculated. The level of change and direction (signed) are specified for each participant. Values are ranked from negative to positive.

The Kruskal-Wallis test is the nonparametric equivalent of the one-way independent group ANOVA. This test is used to test for differences among three or more independent groups. Statistical calculations are similar to the Mann-Whitney U and Wilcoxon rank sum test. The raw data are collected, ranked, and then summed. The test statistics (Mann-Whitney U, Wilcoxon, and z score) are used to determine if there are significant differences between the groups.

If data are ordinal, Spearman's rho may be calculated. This statistic describes the extent and direction of a relationship when variables under consideration are rank ordered. A caregiver interested in examining the relationship between infants' comfort (somewhat comfortable, moderately comfortable, and very comfortable) and gestational age could use this statistical test to establish a correlation. This test is also advisable if data are interval but severely skewed or if the data contain outliers. Kendall's tau is another test similar to Spearman's rho that can be used with ordinal-level data.

Logistic regression is used to predict the likelihood of an event occurring based on a known factor. In this case, the dependent variable is nominal, and the independent (predictor) variable may be nominal-, interval-, or ratio-level data.

▶ Descriptive Statistics

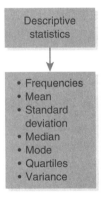

Descriptive statistics are used to describe and synthesize data. Using descriptive statistics, a data set can be described by the shape of the distribution of values (a frequency distribution), measures of central tendency, or the variability of data points. Descriptive statistics are often used in combination with inferential statistics, but they may be used alone.

Frequency Distribution

A frequency distribution displays the frequency of specific outcomes in a sample. To develop a frequency distribution, data points are arranged from the lowest to the highest. How often those data points occur is also identified. Either a table or a graph can be constructed in order to convey the information. For example, the sum of all frequencies equals the N, and the sum of all percentages equals 100.

The same data can also be presented graphically. A histogram can be developed by arranging values horizontally, with the lowest value on the left increasing to the highest value on the right, and displaying frequencies or percentages vertically. Distributions are symmetric if, when they are folded, the two halves are superimposed on one another. In skewed or asymmetric distributions, the peak is not in center.

A tail pointed to the right is positively skewed; a tail to the left is negatively skewed. A frequency distribution and a histogram are presented in **TABLE 6-3** and **FIGURE 6-4**, respectively. Data from a published study (Bugajski et al., 2016) was used to construct Table 6-3 and Figure 6-4 (see **BOX 6-15**).

Calculating a mean (average), median (midpoint), or mode (most frequent) is another approach to reporting descriptive statistics. While the mean of a set of scores

TABLE 6-3 Frequency Table of Total Scores for the BHHRFA

Case Identifier	Frequency	Percent	Valid Percent	Cumulative Percent
0	188	3.2	3.2	3.2
1	550	9.3	9.3	12.5
2	714	12.1	12.1	24.0
3	343	5.8	5.8	30.4
4	306	5.2	5.2	35.5
5	179	3.0	3.0	38.6
6	178	3.0	3.0	41.6
7	123	2.1	2.1	43.7
8	170	2.9	2.9	46.5
9	160	2.7	2.7	49.3
10	162	2.7	2.7	52.0
11	147	2.5	2.5	54.5
12	217	3.7	3.7	58.2
13	208	3.5	3.5	61.7
14	258	4.4	4.4	66.0
15	226	3.8	3.8	69.9
16	228	3.9	3.9	73.7

(continues)

TABLE 6-3 Frequency Table of Total Scores for the BHHRFA				*(continued)*
Case Identifier	**Frequency**	**Percent**	**Valid Percent**	**Cumulative Percent**
17	189	3.2	3.2	76.9
18	215	3.6	3.6	80.6
19	157	2.7	2.7	83.2
20	192	3.2	3.2	86.5
21	223	3.8	3.8	90.2
22	194	3.3	3.3	93.5
23	134	2.3	2.3	95.8
24	85	1.4	1.4	97.2
25	62	1.0	1.0	98.3
26	38	0.6	0.6	98.9
27	19	0.3	0.3	99.2
28	18	0.3	0.3	99.5
29	15	0.3	0.3	99.8
30	5	0.1	0.1	99.9
31	3	0.1	0.1	99.9
32	1	0.0	0.0	99.9
33	1	0.0	0.0	100.0
34	1	0.0	0.0	100.0
35	1	0.0	0.0	100.0
Total	5,910	100.0	100.0	

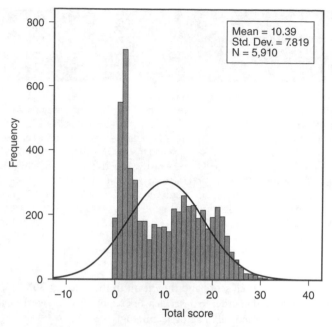

FIGURE 6-4 Histogram for total scores for the BHHRFA.

👥 **BOX 6-15** Drew Bugajski, RN, BSN: Exploring Causes for Increased Incidences of Inpatient Falls on a Psychiatric Unit

Drew conducted a secondary data analysis to discover if the Baptist Health High Risk Falls Assessment (BHHRFA) could predict inpatient falls on a psychiatric inpatient unit. During his data analysis, he first had to analyze the frequencies and distribution of the BHHRFA total scores in both the normal inpatient population and the psychiatric inpatient population. The frequency table (Table 6-3) allowed Drew to see how many entries were recorded for each possible BHHRFA score. He constructed a histogram to graphically display the data and determine if the data were normally distributed (Figure 6-4). The histogram is a series of bars that represent the frequency distribution of each of the BHHRFA scores. Checking the frequencies and viewing the histogram were the first steps Drew took before pursuing further data analysis.

conveys important information, that value does not address the dispersion of scores. For example, if pain scores are calculated using a 0 to 10 scale, 5 may be the mean of two different samples of patients. However, scores of 4s and 5s may have led to a mean of 5 in one sample while scores of 1s and 9s may be responsible for the mean in the other sample.

In relation to pain scores, caregivers may want to understand how many patients are having extreme pain as opposed to others whose pain scores are grouped around the mean (5). Calculating a standard deviation enables investigators to understand the dispersion of their scores. A standard deviation indicates the average amount that scores deviate from the mean. The amount of deviation is captured by calculating

BOX 6-16 Allison Fultz, MBA, RT: Job Satisfaction of Medical Imaging Technologists: A Current Look at Work Environment, Communication, and Leadership

The purpose of this study was to explore factors related to medical imaging technologists' job satisfaction. A 12-item, 3-subscale, investigator-designed questionnaire was used to assess job satisfaction. A total score ranging from 4 to 48 was possible. Education was a factor of interest; investigators examined the differences in responses between technologists who had an associate's degree and those who had a baccalaureate degree. There was no significant difference between the two groups on total job satisfaction (t[39]=−0.067, p=0.947). The mean and standard deviation of the first group were 39.24 and 5.46, respectively; from the second group, the mean was 39.35 and the SD was 5.23. The means and standard deviations of both groups were similar. The average distance from each mean was approximately 5 points. Findings have been accepted for publication in the journal *Radiologic Technology*.

the difference between each score and the mean. In the study in **BOX 6-16**, standard deviations are calculated in order to describe work experience and work environment subscale scores among medical imaging technologists.

▶ Chapter Summary

This chapter was designed to provide sufficient information regarding statistical analysis to enable a caregiver without research experience to feel comfortable addressing the statistical component of the research process. Explanations and definitions of statistical concepts may assist caregivers to better understand the analyses they conduct. An understanding of these concepts may also assist them in developing publishable manuscripts. In this RFE, the purpose of a study, desired outcomes, levels of measurement required by different statistical tests, and underlying principles of tests are considered important information for caregivers to understand prior to conducting research. The requirement in this RFE is not for caregivers to understand specific formulas or mathematical calculations but how to select a particular statistical test and the interpretation of the test.

Consultants pay particular attention to statistical analysis. When reviewing manuscripts prior to submission, they frequently find that authors do not appear to understand the analysis of their data. The data analysis section of their submissions does not clearly fit with the remainder of the article. It is therefore important that authors of manuscript submissions work closely with the consultant that calculated the data analysis so that they clearly understand how data are analyzed and reported.

References

American Nurses Credentialing Center. (2013). In text reference. *2014 Magnet Application Manual*. Silver Springs, MD.

Bugajski, A., Lengerich, A., Marchese, M., Hall, B., Yackzan, S., Davies, C., & Brockopp, D. (2017). The importance of factors related to nurse retention: Using the Baptist Health Nurse

Retention Questionnaire, Part 2. *Journal of Nursing Administration, 47*(6), 308–312. doi:10.1097 /nna.0000000000000486

Bugajski, A., Lengerich, A., McCowan, D., Merritt, S., Moe, K., Hall, B, Nelson, D., . . . , Brockopp, D. (2017). The Baptist Health High-Risk Falls Assessment: One assessment fits all. *Journal of Nursing Care and Quality, 32*(2), 114–119. doi:10.1097/ncq.0000000000000220

Corley, D., Brockopp, D., McCowan, D., Merritt, S., Cobb, T., Johnson, B., . . . , Hall, B. (2014). The Baptist Health High Risk Falls Assessment: A methodological study. *Journal of Nursing Administration, 44*(5), 263–269.

Davies, C., Brockopp, D., & Moe, K. (2015). Test-retest and internal consistency of the Disability of Arm, Shoulder and Hand (DASH) outcome measure in assessing functional status among breast cancer survivors with lymphedema. *Rehabilitation Oncology, 33*(1), 28–31. doi:10.1097 /ncc.0000000000000413

Field, A. P. (2009). *Discovering statistics using SPSS*. London, England: SAGE.

Fultz, A., Walker, M., Lengerich A., & Bugajski, A. (2018). Radiologic technologists' job satisfaction. *Radiologic Technology, 89*(6), 536-540.

Honaker, J. S., Forston, M. R., Davis, E. A., Wiesner, M. M., & Morgan, J. A. (2013). Effects of non-contact low-frequency ultrasound on healing of suspected deep tissue injury: A retrospective analysis. *International Wound Journal, 10*(1), 65–72. doi:10.1111/j.1742-481X.2012.00944.x

Honaker, J., Brockopp, D., & Moe, K. (2014). Development and psychometric testing of the Honaker suspected deep tissue injury severity scale. *Journal of Wound, Ostomy and Continence Nursing, 41*(3), 238–241. doi:10.1097/won.0000000000000024

Kjelland, K., Corley, D., Slusher, I., Moe, K., & Brockopp, D. (2014). The Best for Baby Card: An evaluation of factors that influence women's decisions to breastfeed. *Newborn & Infant Nursing Reviews, 14*(1), 23–27. doi:10.1053/j.nainr.2013.12.007

Lewis, D. A., Sanders, L. P., & Brockopp, D. Y. (2011). The effect of three nursing interventions on thermoregulation in low birth weight infants. *Neonatal Network, 30*(3), 160–164. doi:10.1891 /07300832.30.3.160

Lewis, C. P., Corley, D. J., Lake, N., Brockopp, D., & Moe, K. (2015). Overcoming barriers to effective pain management: the use of professionally directed small group discussions. *Pain Management Nursing, 16*(2), 121–127. doi:10.1016/j.pmn.2014.05.002

Moe, K., Brockopp, D., McCowan, D., Merritt, S., & Hall, B. (2015). Major predictors of inpatient falls: a multisite study. *Journal of Nursing Administration, 45*(10), 498–502. doi:10.1097 /nna.0000000000000241

Pallant, J. (2010). *SPSS survival manual: A step by step guide to data analysis using SPSS*. Maidenhead, NY: Open University Press/McGraw-Hill.

Polit, D. F., & Beck, C. T. (2006). *Nursing research: Generating & assessing evidence for nursing practice*. Philadelphia, PA: Lippincott Williams & Wilkins.

Schreiber, J. A., Cantrell, D., Moe, K. A., Hench, J., McKinney, E., Preston Lewis, C., . . . , Brockopp, D. (2014). Improving knowledge, assessment, and attitudes related to pain management: Evaluation of an intervention. *Pain Management Nursing, 15*(2), 474–481. doi:10.1016/j.pmn.2012.12.006

Stoltz, R., Byrd, R., Hench, A. J., Slone, T., Brockopp, D., & Moe, K. (2014). Does the type of sleep surface influence infant wellbeing in the NICU? *American Journal of Maternal Child Nursing, 39*(6), 363–368. doi:10.1097/nmc.0000000000000078

Winner-Stoltz, R., Lengerich, A., Hench, A., O'Malley, J., Kjelland, K., & Teal, M. Staff nurse perceptions of open pod and single family room NICU designs on work environment and patient care. *Advances in Neonatal Care*, 18(3), 189–198. doi: 10.1097/ANC.0000000000000493

Tabachnick, B. G., & Fidell, L. S. (2007). *Using multivariate statistics* (5th ed.). Boston, MA: Pearson.

Thompson, M., Moe, K., & Lewis, C. P. (2014). The effects of music on diminishing anxiety among preoperative patients. *Journal of Radiology Nursing, 33*(4), 199–202. doi:10.1016/j.jradnu.2014.10.005

Workman, C., Ogle, K., & Lengerich, A. (2017). Differences in quality of life and functional status between two types of procedural anesthesia. Unpublished manuscript.

Weyl, H., Yackzan, S., Ross, K., Henson, A., Moe, K., & Lewis, C. P. (2015). Understanding colorectal screening behaviors and factors associated with screening in a community hospital setting. *Clinical Journal of Oncology Nursing, 19*(1), 89–93. doi:10.1188/15.cjon.89-93

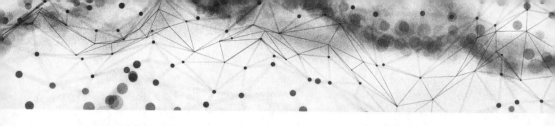

CHAPTER 7
Disseminating Findings

"The critical consumer of research is interested in weighing the strengths and weaknesses of a report and determining the overall usability of findings from an investigation."

—**Brockopp & Hastings-Tolsma**, 2003

▶ Introduction

Disseminating findings is particularly important in a rapidly changing healthcare environment. Caregivers, patients, and hospital administrators can benefit from the findings of caregiver-initiated research. Study results may be used to modify work situations for caregivers, change clinical practice, or motivate investigators to conduct additional studies to increase understanding of a particular problem or issue. Appreciation for caregivers' involvement in research can vary. In this research-friendly environment (RFE), the Board of Trustees recently sent letters to all authors and coauthors of publications thanking them for their commitment to patient care and their dedication to improving practice through conducting research.

There are several assumptions underlying the goal in this RFE to disseminate findings of caregivers' research. The first and probably the most important assumption is related to who can conduct research. The belief that caregivers at the bedside or in administrative roles (regardless of educational preparation) have the ability, with assistance, to conduct research is necessary if hospital administrators are interested in developing an RFE. These same caregivers can also present and/or publish their findings. The assumption that caregivers can write for publication has taken time to become a reality but is now generally accepted throughout this institution.

At a practical level, there is the assumption that hospital administrators support the conduct of research and the dissemination of project results. Given the imperative to base practice on evidence, administrators may need to be increasingly involved in supporting research activities. Sharing results of these activities across institutions can improve patient care for a larger population, enhance the reputation of the institution, and increase job satisfaction for employees.

It is also assumed in a Magnet-designated hospital, or a hospital seeking designation, that supporting nurses to be actively involved in research is a priority. Given that Magnet designation requires nurses at the bedside to be actively involved in research activities, encouraging nurses to present or publish their findings is a logical step at the conclusion of their studies.

Another assumption in this RFE is that caregivers, in general, want to provide optimal patient care. Nurses in particular are influenced by the care provided in their work setting. This assumption in relation to nurses is based on retention data. Nurses want to work in settings that enable them to provide the best care possible (Bugajski et al., 2017). Working in an environment that encourages caregivers to ask questions and resolve patient care problems by conducting research conveys an important message regarding patient care. The message is clear that an ongoing attempt to provide optimal care is inherent to the culture.

Ten years of experience in this RFE also supports the notion that many caregivers are committed to improving patient care. In this institution, an average of 35 to 40 projects initiated by caregivers are ongoing at any one time. Many projects take more than a year to complete. Each year, the results of approximately 8 to 10 projects are thought to be appropriate for publication. Consultants may assist investigators of these projects to write abstracts to submit for a conference presentation, reports for internal use, or manuscripts to submit for publication. In each case, consultants provide face-to-face assistance with writing and, as needed, guide PowerPoint development for presentations to assure accuracy and clarity.

While help is available for abstracts and internal reports, in terms of dissemination, the greatest time and energy expenditure for research consultants is spent preparing manuscripts. Approximately 90% of studies designed with publication as a goal are submitted for publication. Given limited funds for travel to conferences and a desire to disseminate findings, publication of projects is emphasized and encouraged.

Unless it is clear that a project is for internal use only, or a caregiver's goal is to present at a conference, research consultants introduce the possibility of publication in their initial conversations with investigators. Consultants address issues related to potential publication such as the investigator's desire to publish, prior research on the topic, rigor of the proposed study, roles of the principal investigator and co-investigators, and available opportunities for publication.

There are in-hospital benefits related to publishing the findings of caregivers' studies. As the chief nursing officer (CNO) and the librarian announce publications by clinicians throughout the institution, other employees at all levels, including medical staff, become more confident in their ability to also conduct research and publish findings. Requests for consultation from the research office have increased as the number of publications has increased. From an administrative perspective, publications validate the work of the research office. Publications also reflect caregivers' interest in basing clinical practice on evidence.

Using the guidelines presented below, 96% of manuscripts (N=45, over 2011–2018) submitted from this RFE have been accepted for publication. An approach developed in this RFE to assisting caregivers to write manuscripts for submission to a peer-reviewed journal is described in this chapter. This approach differs considerably from the guidance generally provided in academia, as it was designed for use with full-time hospital-based employees.

In addition, a description of the kind and extent of assistance consultants provide to caregivers as they develop a manuscript is presented. The process of review once the manuscript is submitted is described as well, and steps that occur at the journal level are addressed.

▶ Disseminating Findings: The Research Consultant's Role

Typically, caregivers who need to collect and analyze data related to a specific issue that will be addressed internally and will not be disseminated outside of the hospital come to the research office for help with their data. Consultants frequently design a database, assist caregivers to enter and analyze their data, and help them to write a report for internal use. On occasion, these internal reports have led to the design of a study.

Assisting caregivers to write abstracts is more challenging than assisting them to write internal reports. Guidelines for submission of an abstract need to be carefully assessed and followed. A frequent mistake made by caregivers in this RFE, in relation to abstract writing for either a presentation or publication, is not paying sufficient attention to submission requirements. The process is different from caregivers' usual activities and as such presents a challenge. Meeting that challenge requires consultants to provide guidance and impart information. Building caregivers' confidence on a continuous basis is also important. Teaching includes helping caregivers to write in a particular manner, learn words and phrases that are part of the research process, and understand statistical analysis.

The steps presented below evolved over 10 years of experience in this RFE mentoring caregivers who needed assistance with data in order to write an internal report, needed help writing an abstract, or wanted to conduct research and publish their findings. The process is designed to assist hospital-based caregivers to take their clinical experience, transform that experience into a search for evidence to support practice change, and disseminate their results. Although consultants may be involved in all aspects of evaluating practice, transforming practice into publication is a major goal of research activities in this RFE (Brockopp, Hill, Moe, & Wright, 2016).

Internal Reports

Research consultant activities focused on outcomes internal to the institution have ranged from developing a questionnaire for a physician who wanted to assess attitudes among members of a large multisite committee to helping the Director of Case Management collect information regarding reasons why patients are readmitted to the hospital within 30 days of discharge. An example of assisting a caregiver with an internal report is presented in **BOX 7-1**.

Abstracts

Abstracts, whether written for the beginning of an article or submission for presentation at a conference, are similar in terms of requirements. Regardless of the

BOX 7-1 Denise McCowan, RN, MSN: Reasons for Patient Thirty-Day Readmissions

Denise was asked by administration to examine potential reasons for patient readmissions to the hospital within 30 days. The purpose of this project was to provide administration with information that could be used to diminish the number of readmissions within this time period. A research consultant assisted with the development of a questionnaire and designed a database. Case managers input the data. The consultant analyzed the data and constructed a preliminary report that was shared with the director. Her sample (N=98) included 37 men (37.8%) and 61 women (62.2%). The payment source for the largest group was Medicare (N=47, 48%), and the first admission diagnosis for 77 (78.6%) patients was illness rather than a surgery/procedure. Regarding their prior admission, most patients (N=83, 91.2%) felt ready to be discharged, 53 (84.1%) felt their symptoms worsening, and 44 (57.9%) patients contacted someone to help them before returning to the hospital. Findings were reported to administration. (Permission was granted to include findings in this text.)

TABLE 7-1 Guidance for Submitting Abstracts

Goals or purpose of presentation/project	Explain clearly and concisely the issue addressed and the context of the project or presentation
Importance	Describe the relevance of the project to the audience
Methods	Detail methods: Background, design, measures, sample, data analysis, and results
Findings	Provide a clear description of results of statistical analysis
Conclusion/Summary	Describe possible changes that could be introduced based on findings. In addition, suggestions for future research are often welcomed.

purpose, abstracts need to follow guidelines provided by the journal or conference administrators. Headings, formatting, and word count are often specified. In addition, understanding the importance of flow, formatting and specified headings is an essential first step for a novice author.

When responding to a call for abstracts, authors need to ensure that the research question reflects the goals of the conference and the interests of the audience. When a study is conducted within a hospital setting, caregivers may be required to obtain permission to present findings regarding data collected at that institution. Permission is essential if hospital proprietary data are included in the presentation. **TABLE 7-1** provides guidance for caregivers submitting abstracts for presentation at a conference. Approval of administration prior to submission of abstracts for presentation at a conference or manuscript submissions is highly recommended.

When an abstract has been accepted for presentation (verbal or poster), research consultants often critique caregivers' presentations. Problems with presentations may

BOX 7-2 Sarah Groppo-Lawless, MS, CCC, SLP: Screening for Dysphagia

Sarah was concerned about early identification of dysphagia among hospitalized patients diagnosed with pneumonia. She wanted to develop a tool that nurses could use to screen for dysphagia among patients admitted with a diagnosis of pneumonia, as a standardized nurse dysphagia screening tool for this patient population was not available. Such a screen would enable early identification of patients at risk for dysphagia and referral to a speech-language pathologist. She worked with consultants to design a two-phase study. In Phase 1, she assessed inpatients (N=301) diagnosed with pneumonia for 25 risk factors for dysphagia. In Phase 2, she selected the most prevalent risk factors among the 25 factors by assessing risk factors among patients (N=129) who failed a 3-ounce water trial.

The conference submission form required Sarah to include her present position, professional affiliations, certifications, a brief biographical sketch, her choice of verbal or poster presentation, learner outcomes, and an abstract of her work with references. Her work was accepted for a poster presentation. Following her presentation, Sarah tested her assessment for predictive validity on patients diagnosed with pneumonia (N=178) and submitted her findings for publication (Groppo-Lawless, Bugajski, & Lengerich, 2018).

include poor adherence to time allotted, lack of clarity of PowerPoint slides, and/or omission of important components of statistical analyses. To help caregivers be as successful as possible, presenters at the annual research symposium in this RFE are required to present to a colleague or consultant before their formal presentation. Consultants will also review presentations by caregivers who have abstracts accepted regionally or nationally.

Research consultants assisted a speech-language pathologist to write and submit an abstract for the Speech-Language-Hearing Association's national convention in 2016. The speech-language pathologist decided to submit her abstract for a poster presentation, and her abstract was subsequently accepted. (See **BOX 7-2**.)

▶ Transforming Practice into Publication: A Research-Friendly Institution's Guide

The steps outlined below were used to assist caregivers to publish the findings of their studies. Out of 48 submissions, only 1 manuscript has been rejected. One manuscript did not require changes, and the remainder were accepted following revisions. Depending on their expertise in the area of research and writing for publication, caregivers who come to the office may need to spend considerable time with consultants or very little time. Approximately 75% of first authors in this RFE had not published previously and therefore spent several hours with consultants.

There are seven steps in this process. Each step is described in detail. Examples of caregiver's studies reflecting the activities involved in the process are presented. This guide exemplifies the basic philosophy of this RFE: the importance of a caregiver's ideas related to improving practice through research is central to conducting research and the process of publication. Research consultants are methodologists who assist caregivers and other hospital employees to reach their goals.

Step 1: Preparing Early for Publication

Clarifying the purpose of a proposed project is part of the first discussion with caregivers as they come to the research office with their ideas. If project results need to remain within the institution, there is no discussion of publication, and consultants help caregivers construct an internal report for dissemination. If a caregiver is initially interested in constructing an abstract for submission to a regional or national conference at the conclusion of their study, consultants encourage them to consider publication as well as presentation. To date, the majority of caregivers have embraced the idea of publishing their findings. They are interested in moving forward with their projects in ways that optimize the possibility of dissemination through publication.

Caregivers, in general, come to the research office with a specific concern or idea related to improving patient care. Consultants ask them to conduct a search of the literature to provide a foundation for their idea. A librarian is available to help them with a search or, if desired, to teach them the skills to search the literature themselves. Working with the results of their search, consultants help caregivers to construct a meaningful and feasible research question. The question is meaningful when it is likely that study results can lead to changes in practice and dissemination through publication. Feasibility is assessed in terms of resources required and participant availability. Caregivers discover, as a result of their literature review, the extent and value of prior research conducted in their area of interest. Following this search and working with consultants, caregivers make a decision regarding the direction of their project.

Given the range of topics investigated in this RFE, the number of studies available on each topic as well as the timeliness of prior research differ greatly. For example, when investigators reviewed the literature related to the effect of massage on neonatal abstinence syndrome (NAS) babies, no one had investigated that particular intervention within that population. The probability of investigators publishing their results was, therefore, strong. Upon completion of their study, their manuscript was accepted with minor revisions, on first submission, to a journal interested in creative approaches to patient care (Hahn et al., 2016).

A different situation occurred when administration proposed developing a study to better understand factors related to nurse retention. Rather than an absence of literature on a topic, there were numerous studies available. Unfortunately, most of the research was 10 or more years old. As a result, factors identified as important to retention, as discovered in the literature, were questionable. That situation required investigators to evaluate changes in the nursing profession that might influence the validity of factors previously identified. Following that assessment, factors that appeared to be more relevant to present circumstances in nursing were included in the development of a retention assessment. Adding up-to-date items to the instrument resulted in a successful study and publication of results (Lengerich et al., 2017).

A third situation occurred in relation to the topic of pain management. A caregiver, for his DNP project, was interested in improving critical care nurses' knowledge and attitudes regarding the management of pain among critically ill patients. Multiple studies were available on the issue of pain management. In his literature review, he found a study that tested a small group discussion intervention (Brockopp et al., 2004). The intervention was used with nurses working on medical-surgical units. He replicated that study in a different setting: critical care. His study was accepted for publication (Lewis, Corley, McCowan, Merritt, & Hall, 2015).

In each case, caregivers used the literature to reach decisions regarding their study design and specific goals. They also considered the potential for publication given their research question. Questions related to how they might improve NAS babies' comfort, retain hospital-based nurses, and provide better pain control for critically ill patients were addressed in ways that would add to the literature.

Trying to publish results of studies when there is no prior research on the topic, when available studies are outdated, or when the literature suggests that most aspects of a topic have been reported can be difficult. However, even though there is no prior research in a particular area, if the proposed project is new and/or innovative, information retrieved can be of major interest to a wide audience regardless of the literature. For example, a group of investigators with an innovative idea, who could find minimal prior research (none in the United States) on their topic of interest, are presently conducting a study that is likely to be accepted for publication. Investigators' discussions with consultants revealed that the number of NAS babies born in the United States is growing exponentially. In addition, there are few interventions presented in the literature that are effective in comforting these infants. These investigators are conducting a study using a creative intervention that has not been applied in this population. That combination of facts suggests that, depending on study outcomes, a manuscript will be accepted for publication. See **BOX 7-3**.

When preparing investigators for the possibility of publishing their findings, another important consideration is authorship. The topic of authorship is discussed early in consultations with caregivers. Frequently, colleagues of primary investigators assist with data collection, input of data, and/or consenting potential participants during recruitment. Because many caregivers at this institution are publishing for the first time, they are frequently unaware that those individuals who help them can and should be coauthors. Discussing coauthorship of a manuscript with colleagues at the beginning of a study diminishes confusion at the time of submission. In addition, it is often a motivator for colleagues to remain involved and pursue research activities of their own at the conclusion of the study. In this RFE, coauthors contribute to the writing/editing of a final manuscript and must approve submission to a journal. An example of an investigator who involved her colleagues early in her study and asked them to be coauthors is presented in **BOX 7-4**.

 BOX 7-3 Jeri Hahn, RN, BSN, CIMI: Effect of Submersion on NAS Babies

Jeri and her colleagues are interested in the well-being of babies experiencing NAS. These babies, born to women with substance use disorder, have a difficult time during the first weeks of life. Having conducted and published a study on the effect of infant massage on these infants' well-being (Hahn et al., 2015), Jeri is now in the process of initiating a study to see if submersing these infants in water for a short period of time will enhance their physical and social well-being. A search of the literature did not reveal any studies using this intervention with these babies. As a result, considerable effort was needed to discover an appropriate tub, design an assessment, and make decisions regarding the process of collecting data. Given the increase in the number of NAS babies born each year and the difficulties faced by caregivers who try to help them, Jeri's study is likely to be published.

> **BOX 7-4** Heather Bradley, RN, MSN: Preceptor Performance: A Methodological Study
>
> Heather developed an instrument to evaluate preceptor performance and proficiency (the Baptist Health Lexington Performance and Proficiency Assessment). Her multisite study (Bradley et al., 2015) was conducted at four hospitals. One research consultant, two staff nurses, three nurse directors, a special projects nurse, and a nurse educator worked with Heather to assist her with various aspects of her project. Data collection, data input, assistance with data analysis, and editing of a final manuscript were carried out by these individuals. The decision was made early in the consultation process to include these eight colleagues along with Heather as authors of the publication.

Step 2: Evaluating Rigor of Design

The randomized controlled trial (RCT) has been described as the most rigorous study design, although, depending on the research question, it is often not appropriate. Both qualitative and quantitative designs have been described along with strengths and weaknesses of each approach.

Rigor, in terms of designing studies in this RFE with the goal of publishing results, refers to the most rigorous application possible, of each study design. Using quantitative methods, there are five commonly used research questions that caregivers consider when they are concerned about a clinical issue:

- To what extent is a dependent variable (e.g., nurses' intent to stay) found in a population of interest (e.g., hospital-based nurses)?
- What is the effect of an independent variable (e.g., music) on a dependent variable (anxiety level) in a population of interest (e.g., patients prior to surgery)?
- What is the difference between one variable (e.g., age) and another variable (e.g., interest in graduate school) in a population of interest (e.g., hospital-based physical therapists)?
- What is the relationship between one variable (e.g., years of nursing experience) and another variable (e.g., satisfaction with career choice) in a population of interest (e.g., outpatient clinic nurses)?
- How well does one variable (e.g., pain level) predict another variable (e.g., functional status) in a population of interest (e.g., patients diagnosed with arthritis)?

Questions constructed for studies using qualitative methods may be similar to questions posed for quantitative studies. Investigators in this RFE who designed qualitative studies asked questions focused on the psychological response of women to mastectomy, NAS babies' response to massage, and NAS babies' response to hydrotherapy. Phenomenological and descriptive qualitative methods were used.

Following the identification of an appropriate research question related to the caregiver's topic of interest, a sequence of activities regarding publication is determined. A guide for working on a publication is discussed with investigators. The following activities are necessary in order to develop a publishable manuscript, and novice investigators are educated in the process. Consultants guide investigators to be certain that they have a clear, well-written synthesis of background information; identified an appropriate sample size, a description of inclusion criteria for the sample, and a

> **BOX 7-5** Judith Schreiber, RN, PhD: Pain Management: Evaluation of an Intervention
>
> Judith, a research consultant at the time, and her research team conducted a study to improve knowledge, assessment, and attitudes related to pain management among nurses (Schreiber et al., 2014). Watson's Theory of Caring was used as the theoretical framework for the study. A synthesis of background information was not difficult given recent available research in the area of pain control. Because the plan was to compare two groups of patients using a t test, a power analysis was conducted to determine an appropriate sample size (patients N=60, 30 in each group). Nurses (N=341) attended a 2-day workshop led by a national pain management expert. A published measure, the Brockopp-Warden Pain Knowledge/Bias Questionnaire, was used. Statistical analyses included t tests, chi-square tests, and descriptive statistics (means, standard deviations, and percentages). Expectations of a quasi-experiment were met, and her manuscript was accepted on first submission.

detailed description of the intervention if indicated; and identified measures to be used. If published measures are not applicable or available, an investigator-designed instrument will be created. Elements of the instrument design process are described in a publication or presentation. Often, a copy of the instrument will be incorporated into the manuscript as supplemental content. Statistical analyses will be reviewed to assure that authors understand how results were achieved. Limitations are identified and presented. An example of this process is provided in **BOX 7-5**.

Step 3: Developing the Manuscript

Following completion of a study, research consultants and investigators revisit the potential for publication of study results. On occasion, additional data may need to be collected in order to develop a strong manuscript for submission. To date, results of all studies completed with publication as an outcome have been submitted for publication. All coauthors, at least one research consultant, and the CNO review manuscripts prior to submission.

A plan for developing a manuscript includes a tentative timeline. The timeline is tentative given the busy and at times unpredictable schedules of caregivers. Prior to writing the manuscript, consultants meet with the principal investigator(s) to discuss a number of important issues. At this time, consultants try to ensure that caregivers understand the statistical analyses of their data, that they understand caregivers' comfort level regarding writing, and that coauthors' roles have been clarified. Based on this discussion, research consultants gain an understanding of the extent of their involvement in the preparation of a manuscript.

Planning for the publication process includes an examination of the time that has elapsed since the initiation of a study. Outcomes of recent studies are considered for addition to the background section of the manuscript. On occasion, recent work can negatively influence chances of publication. For example, an employee enrolled in a graduate program came to the office with a paper she had written for her coursework. Her faculty member recommended that she submit the paper for publication. Unfortunately, the same research question had been addressed and published in the preceding 6 months. The publication was in the journal she had selected as the most

BOX 7-6 Lindsay Bowles, RN, BSN: The Effect of Music on Exercise

Lindsay contacted research consultants for assistance in designing a study to assess the influence of music on exercise among cardiac rehabilitation patients. She and her co-investigators completed the study, data were analyzed, and results reviewed in the research office. She met with a research consultant, and they discussed the development of a manuscript. She decided to submit an abstract to the institution's annual symposium for presentation before working on a publication. The abstract was accepted; she presented her work at the symposium and then came back to the research office for help preparing a manuscript. A flexible timeline was developed. Lindsay had not written a manuscript prior to conducting this study and wanted help to move forward. Her manuscript has been submitted for publication.

appropriate for submission given her topic. Research consultants advised her that it was unlikely that her paper would be accepted for publication.

Although research consultants typically analyze data with the investigator(s) present, there are times when additional consultation regarding the principles of statistical analysis is necessary. A general lack of understanding of the application of statistics among caregivers requires consultants to verify their understanding of analyses conducted using their data. This understanding is not only necessary for the writing of a manuscript but is essential if authors, at some point, present their work to colleagues.

When the possibility of publishing the results of their studies is first discussed, most caregivers in this RFE are concerned about their ability to write for publication. Writing for publication is not an activity they expected to undertake, and they do not feel prepared. Consultants spend considerable effort assuring them of the help that is available and that, like caregivers before them, they can be successful. An example of a caregiver who worked with consultants to submit a manuscript to a peer-reviewed journal is presented in **BOX 7-6**.

Involvement of other individuals in publishing the results of a study is also discussed in early meetings between consultants and caregivers. Even though coauthors were identified at the initiation of a study, primary investigators are sometimes unaware that their coauthors need to edit and approve a final submission.

Step 4: Selecting a Journal

To date, most, if not all, caregivers in this RFE believe that the process of selecting a journal is based on content alone. For example, if studying cardiac issues, caregivers frequently suggest any journal that publishes articles related to heart disease. In some instances, they select the journal that is best known in a given field. Apparently, in many undergraduate and graduate programs, recommendations regarding publication have focused on identifying journals for manuscript submission by content area without consideration of other issues. The problem with this approach is that journals differ across a number of factors, including preferred research design and the rigor of the application of the design. Some journals favor the use of advanced statistics as opposed to basic statistics. Timing of publications, composition of editorial boards, and expectations regarding author credentials are a few additional ways that journals differ.

In terms of research design, an examination of journals that focus on a particular disease category or components of health administration will usually reveal clear preferences for specific research designs. For some journals, most studies published are RCTs; in some cases, all studies published involve quantitative methods. In addition, in some journals, descriptive studies are not published. To increase the likelihood of acceptance of a manuscript, the research design (RCT, quasi-experiment, descriptive design, qualitative design) should match most of the studies published in a given journal.

In addition to research design, how well the design was followed (rigor) and the level of statistical analysis used are factors to consider when selecting a journal. Studies that include the use of advanced statistics as opposed to basic analyses are more prevalent in some journals. In most cases in this RFE, basic statistics (t tests, chi-square, ANOVA, linear/logistic regression) are used to analyze data. A match in this regard may increase the chances of acceptance of a manuscript.

The focus of journals may differ even though they address the same disease category. For example, in oncology there are journals that emphasize research while others are focused on clinical practice. In the area of pain management, some journals reflect an interest in healthcare professionals who deliver anesthesia while others focus on bedside care. Reviewing three or four articles in several different journals can help investigators to select the journal that is most likely to accept their manuscript.

Timing of publication is also important. A journal that publishes quarterly may not accept as many articles for publication as a journal that publishes monthly. Another aspect of timing relates to the length of the review process. If the review process at a given journal takes a year to complete, the results of a study may lose their value if the manuscript is rejected and requires submission to another journal. Some journals are clear in the information they provide regarding the time the review process takes, but others are not.

An interesting component of journal selection has to do with professional affiliations of editorial board members and credentials of authors. It does not appear to be accidental that journals where most or all editorial board members represent one profession publish few articles by individuals outside of that profession. In addition, an examination of journals reveals a tendency to publish manuscripts authored by individuals who have graduate degrees. Given that individuals with both baccalaureate and associate's degrees conduct research in this RFE, authorship credentials are an important factor to assess when selecting a journal. Although some of the questions addressed regarding differences in journals can be addressed with an editor, frequently these patterns are not formal but have evolved over time. Examining these patterns and making choices based on those patterns can increase the likelihood of publication.

How often articles in a particular journal are cited is another factor that might influence selection of a journal. The Journal Citation Reports (Minnick, 2017) provides information on tools for ranking, evaluating, categorizing, and comparing journals with editorial metrics. The impact factor—that is, the number of times a journal article is cited by other journals—is reported for the previous 2 years. Other indicators known as altmetric indicators may also be relevant when selecting a journal for publication. Altmetric indicators reflect the attention the research in a targeted journal receives from social media. These indicators are often reported on a journal website.

An example of the process of selecting a journal involved a hospital administrator in this RFE. She participated in the planning for the addition of a bed tower to the present hospital campus. She was responsible for the actual move, and with the help of research consultants, she prepared a manuscript for publication. Initially, she

BOX 7-7 Kathy Tussey, MSN, RN: A Move to A Bed Tower—An Evaluation

Kathy, with the help of a consultant, planned to submit a manuscript describing her experience guiding a major move to a bed tower to a journal that publishes clinical opinion articles. Following the outline used in the journal, Kathy and the consultant developed headings of design, timeline, budget, planning for the move, education, move day, evaluation, and summary. On completion of the draft, some additional data became available related to the move. Data on nurse satisfaction with the new environment in the neonatal intensive care unit as well as overall nurse satisfaction collected through an agency contract with the hospital strengthened the manuscript in the direction of evaluation rather than description of events. Based on the availability of these new data, Kathy and the consultants decided to select a journal that publishes data-based articles. After selecting a different journal, Kathy and the consultant revisited the process. Using articles from the journal as a guide, headings were changed, sections rewritten, tables added, and a draft completed (Tussey, Yackzan, & Davies, 2018).

included limited data evaluating staff satisfaction. The manuscript focused largely on a description of the move process. As more data became available, her journal selection changed. See **BOX 7-7**.

Step 5: Collaborative Writing

The goal of research consultants is to assist investigators to develop a manuscript that is clearly and concisely written. Research terms are used as appropriate, and statistical analysis is presented in an understandable manner. Engaging the reader is important, and presenting accurate information is essential. To engage readers, consultants help investigators to present their topic using words and phrases that will interest the audience. Clear and concise writing is accomplished by providing one-on-one assistance.

Once a journal is selected, investigators are asked to bring three or four articles from that journal to consultants in the research office. The content of these articles does not need to reflect the content of the caregiver's study, as these articles are used as models. They are reviewed for style of writing; use of first person (or not); length of each section (e.g., background, measures, discussion); headings used; and extent of detail provided in statistical analysis component, discussion, and conclusion. An outline using these characteristics is developed.

This assistance includes both developing an outline and constructing sentences as needed. The outline is based on the three or four articles obtained from the target journal. Investigators who have not written for some time often need help to get started. Sitting together with new investigators to write the first few sentences is often helpful. Asking new authors to bring bulleted points of content that are most important to the investigator often assists them to begin the writing process.

Initially, as a part of the writing process, consultants work with investigators to ensure that the original research question is clearly articulated. The remainder of the manuscript flows from that question (or statement). The institutional review board application contains descriptions of sample, measures, rationale for the study, and proposed methods of analysis. It is often helpful to have that document, along with the three or four articles from the target journal, present as consultants and investigators begin the process of developing a manuscript.

New authors are often unaware of the importance of accuracy when reporting results. They learn, working with consultants, that each statistical test used in data analysis must be presented and clearly described. Research language, particularly words, phrases, and symbols used in statistical analyses, is frequently a problem for new authors. Consultants often write the statistical section of a manuscript; however, that section is discussed thoroughly with investigators. Changes in writing to match the author's style can be made.

In addition, for new authors, writing so that one section of a manuscript flows clearly to the next can be problematic. In this regard, the discussion section frequently is the most difficult for caregivers to complete. Given that some latitude in discussing results is available, wandering from the topic studied does occur. Asking caregivers to bullet point those ideas they want in the discussion section can be helpful. Once organized, those bullet points can readily be translated into paragraphs.

Writing in the third person, for those journals that do not accept manuscripts written in the first person, can also be problematic. Caregivers may be unaccustomed to writing in the third person. Working with consultants, they learn how to incorporate words and phrases using the third person rather than the first. Author guidelines are also addressed. Requirements for margins, font size, and number of words for specific sections of the manuscript are carefully reviewed in the manuscript.

As investigators gain confidence in their ability to write, they work independently. Even so, suggestions for changes in their drafts are made in person. The experience in this RFE is that caregivers are more willing to attempt to write a manuscript with one-on-one, face-to-face support than receiving documents with track changes. In addition, they appear to learn more rapidly using this approach. Because the extent of writing assistance provided in this RFE goes beyond exchanging comments electronically, caregivers report that the personal experience is more enjoyable. Anecdotally, new authors have conveyed to research consultants their reluctance to write a manuscript without one-on-one interaction and support.

When assisting caregivers to write for publication, their professional responsibilities, as well as work schedules, are considerations. Hospital-based caregivers' work lives tend to be demanding. For that reason, approaches that can motivate them to publish their work and make the time to write have been developed. For example, collaborating in person with caregivers can diminish procrastination, enhance satisfaction with the process of writing, and encourage future research activities. An example of collaborative writing with an investigator is presented in **BOX 7-8**.

Step 6: Journal Submission

Depending on the journal, submission of a manuscript can involve a number of steps. Assisting caregivers with the process helps them to learn these steps and prepare them for subsequent submissions. First steps include checking for adherence to author guidelines and obtaining coauthor permissions. Often, investigators do not realize that permission from coauthors needs to be obtained and submitted to the journal. A letter of introduction to the journal is also written. Consultants do not submit caregivers' manuscripts—they sit with investigators and assist them to complete the process.

BOX 7-8 Debra Lewis, RN, BSN: The Effect of Three Nursing Interventions on Thermoregulation in Low-Birthweight Infants

Debra's study examining occlusive wrap, chemical mattress, and regulation of room temperature on thermoregulation among low-birthweight infants (N=67) was accepted for publication with minor revisions on first submission (Lewis, Sanders, & Brockopp, 2011). Debra had not developed a manuscript for publication prior to conducting her study. She worked collaboratively with a research consultant to identify an appropriate journal and select three articles to use as models. Debra wrote the first sentence, "From the earliest days of swaddling an infant to the invention of the incubator in the late 1800s, hypothermia among low birth weight (LBW) infants has been a concern" (Lewis, Sanders, & Brockopp, 2011). She and the consultant discussed other ideas for the background, and Debra continued to write. The typical length of the background and other sections in the journal articles were considered. Headings were developed and bullet points written. Debra would leave the office and continue to write. Regular meetings were held to review and edit the manuscript. Prior to submission, colleagues and consultants who had not worked on the manuscript edited the final draft and offered suggestions.

TABLE 7-2 Response to Request for Revisions

Title of Article:		
Journal:		
Date Received:		

Revision	**Page No.**	**Response to Revision**
Revision #1		Response #1
Revision #2		Response #2
Revision #3		Response #3

Step 7: Response to Request for Revisions

It is rare in the experience in this RFE to have articles accepted for publication without a request for revision. For the most part, revisions are minor, but occasionally, major revisions are requested. In order to respond in a clear, understandable manner, revisions are sent to journal editors using the form shown in **TABLE 7-2**.

At times, under response to revisions, suggested changes are not made. Instead, a rationale for why the original statement or idea was included is presented. A reviewer may not be aware of the accuracy of a given statement; in that case, the author will work with a consultant to find evidence for the particular idea or statement. He or she will provide a reason for including the statement as well as a reference supporting that inclusion.

Unfortunately, not all reviews of manuscripts are productive. At times, it appears that reviewers have not carefully evaluated all components of a manuscript. Reviewers may also convey a personal, negative bias toward the topic studied. To avoid a negative experience for new authors, consultants urge authors to bring their reviews to the research office before addressing the issues raised. Consultants help new authors assess reviews and understand that while most comments will be meaningful, others may not.

Transforming Practice into Publication: A Research-Friendly Environment's Guide: Summary

Using these steps, consultants have assisted caregivers to publish numerous manuscripts over a 10-year period. Over this timeframe, changes in attitudes, such as those regarding who should publish, have occurred. Two nurses prepared at the associate-degree level, with little experience in research, have conducted clinically useful studies and published their findings in peer-reviewed journals. These individuals have set the stage for caregivers with varying backgrounds to do the same. They are examples of the philosophical foundation of this RFE, which supports the notion that the clinical expertise and creativity of the caregiver are most important. Consultants provide the methods for caregivers to improve practice.

Knowledge regarding the extent and kind of assistance available to caregivers who want to publish their research findings has spread throughout the institution. Similarly, observing caregivers' success in publishing manuscripts has convinced others to do the same. New authors continually express their gratitude for consultants' assistance with their projects. Perhaps the different approach to providing assistance with an "academic" activity is responsible.

Outcomes of conducting research and publishing findings often include returning to school. To date, 13% of authors have returned to school seeking advanced degrees. Interest in roles that include a major component in evaluation has also increased. The desire of caregivers to remain at this institution has also been conveyed anecdotally to research consultants. They speak to the importance of having the resources and support to advance themselves intellectually and personally.

▶ Disseminating Findings: The Journal's Perspective

Steps 1 through 7, identified in this chapter, describe a process to assist hospital-based caregivers to develop a manuscript for submission to a peer-reviewed journal. Peer review is a process wherein professional peers (two or more) evaluate a manuscript and comment on the presentation and content. Another process occurs as the editor of a journal receives a manuscript for review. An understanding of this process can be helpful as caregivers are preparing their submission. **FIGURE 7-1** describes a typical process that occurs following submission of a manuscript to the editor of a peer-reviewed journal.

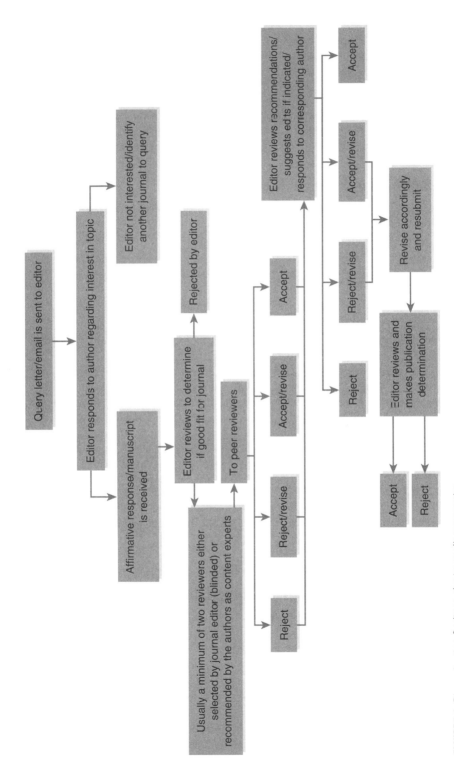

FIGURE 7-1 Disseminating findings: the journal's perspective.

> **BOX 7-9** Letter to the Editor
>
> **Dear Editor,**
> My name is Joan Smith and I am the Chief Nursing Officer at Sunset Health. I have been working on a project with my team to explore the relationship between the performance of bedside report and the incidence of falls with injury on a medical-surgical unit. My team has conducted a project looking at the impact on our fall rate since we implemented bedside report over a year ago. The project was approved by our institutional review board and is showing meaningful results. We feel that this study and the findings will be of interest to your readers. We expect to have our manuscript ready to submit by May 1. Can you please let us know if you think this is a good fit for your journal? We have also reviewed the Guidelines for Authors available on your web site.
>
> Our team is comprised of clinical nurse experts, a physical therapist, and an administrative lead, all with many years of nursing experience. Thank you for your consideration of this possible submission.
>
> Sincerely,
> Joan Smith, DNP, RN, NEA-BC
> Chief Nursing Officer

Letter or Email Message Is Sent to the Editor

Editors often receive inquiries regarding the appropriateness of a manuscript for a particular journal. When there is a concern about appropriate fit of a manuscript with a particular journal, consultants recommend that investigators send a letter to the editor. The letter usually includes a brief description of the topic and an outline of methods used to conduct their project. An example of a letter is presented in **BOX 7-9**.

Editor Responds to an Inquiry

Editors will respond to authors with their interest or lack thereof in reviewing a manuscript. When responding to authors, some editors will suggest a different journal that may be more appropriate for a particular submission. If an editor is interested in a manuscript, authors have completed the first step toward publication. An editor's agreement to read a submission, however, does not imply that the manuscript will move further through the process. This step simply means that the editor will read the manuscript and make a decision as whether or not it will move forward for peer review.

Editor's Decision to Reject or Forward for Review

Editors will review manuscripts preceded by a letter of inquiry or manuscripts sent directly to them without an introduction. They assess the content, format, and overall presentation in relation to expectations of articles published in their journals. Problems may include the following: topic does not reflect interests of the journal (a letter of inquiry may have been misleading), nonadherence to author guidelines, and absence of permissions from coauthors. Additional permissions from hospitals may also be missing. Administrators need to agree in writing that the name of the organization can be featured in a publication and that the data collected and analyzed are acceptable to them.

In addition, potential copyright issues may be a barrier. For example, if an author refers to a published model and includes a schematic of that model, he or she may need permission from the publisher to include it in a manuscript. Attending to all of the details required for a submission enhances chances of the manuscript going forward for peer review.

Role of Peer Reviewers

Editors of some journals ask authors to provide names of individuals who have expertise in the particular area of research described in the manuscript to act as peer reviewers. Other editors, although they do not customarily ask for names of experts in a particular area, respond positively to an author's request to have a specific individual with expertise in the area studied to review a submission. The policy at most journals, however, is to require a blind review. In the case of a blind review, the reviewer is unknown to the author. Many editors agree that a blind review is the most objective approach to peer reviews.

Reviewers for journals may have expertise in methods such as psychometrics, statistics, and/or the particular area under study. Expertise in writing and the research process are general requirements. The number of reviewers assigned to a manuscript can vary; however, two is usually the minimum number assigned. At times, as necessary, the editor may serve as a reviewer making the final decision of acceptance or rejection.

Response to Authors: Editors and Reviewers

There are four responses that editors and reviewers can make to authors. They may reject the manuscript, reject it with the recommendation that authors revise their work, accept the manuscript with revisions, or accept it without revisions. Depending on the journal, suggestions from reviewers may range from extremely to not particularly helpful. In general, editors and reviewers expect authors to respond carefully and in detail to all comments related to their submission, regardless of the helpfulness of those comments. An example of a method used in this RFE to respond to reviewers' recommendations is described in Table 7-1. Other methods could be equally as successful in obtaining acceptance of a manuscript as long as each of the reviewers' comments is thoughtfully addressed.

Requests for Revisions

Characteristics of a manuscript that cause reviewers to request revisions include writing not up to the standard of the journal, data not adequately presented, sections not flowing in a logical sequence, statistical analysis not fitting with prior content, and an inadequate conclusion. When a number of these characteristics occur in the same manuscript, it may be rejected without recommending revisions.

Writing that is clear, understandable, and engaging is a major factor in the acceptance of a manuscript for publication. Synthesizing material, citing important ideas, and leaving the reader with a clear understanding of both methods and outcomes are keys to success. Assisting authors to improve a poorly written manuscript is probably the most challenging task facing reviewers. If sentences are poorly constructed and grammar is incorrect, it is likely the manuscript will be rejected.

In terms of data presentation, data must be complete and accurate. The processes of data collection analysis need to be easily understood. Problems occur when data collected do not match data used in the statistical analyses described in the manuscript. Another problem occurs when mathematical steps are taken that are inaccurate. For example, the number of participants in a study may change. In phase 1 of a study, there are 50 participants, but by phase 2, some participants may drop out of the study. It is not acceptable to simply change the number of participants in the analysis section without identifying the fact that a certain number of participants are no longer enrolled.

Occasionally, content in an abstract of a manuscript will differ from what is presented under data analysis and conclusions. In addition, what is written in the background section may deviate from the focus of the study. When sections of a manuscript do not logically flow from research question to conclusion, either the manuscript is rejected or revisions are requested.

At times, it is apparent to reviewers that individuals with statistical expertise have written the data analysis section of a manuscript. While that may be appropriate, the remainder of the manuscript needs to relate to the analysis of data. On occasion, the writing style is different in the statistical analysis section, the content prior to the analysis section may not flow appropriately into the analyses, and the discussion section does not accurately reflect results of the analysis. Authors' understanding of statistical analyses of their data can prevent this problem. The logical sequencing of sections of a manuscript from abstract to conclusion is probably the most important characteristic of a strong submission.

▶ Chapter Summary

Dealing with a changing healthcare environment necessitates resolving patient care problems on a continuous basis. Experienced caregivers are particularly skilled at identifying problems and often suggesting alternative approaches to care. Given their experience at the bedside, they have the ability to construct exciting research questions. With assistance, they can conduct studies and disseminate their findings. As a result, caregiver-initiated research can provide information that will improve patient care in their own institution and across settings.

The model proposed in this chapter is based on assumptions that differ to some extent from a traditional view of hospital-based research and publication. Caregivers who want to improve practice and have ideas regarding how practice could be changed come to the research office. They are, to a great extent, embarking on an unknown journey. Frequently, they come with an understanding that a lack of research skills may prevent them from conducting a study. In reality, little or no prior experience in research or a lack of credentials suggesting the presence of research skills is not a deterrent.

This traditional approach to research supports the notion that PhD-prepared healthcare professionals design and conduct studies necessary to base patient care on evidence. The individual with a PhD is the primary investigator of each study conducted and first author on publications. In some circumstances, caregivers at the bedside may be coauthors. In this model, it would seem that research skills are of greater importance than content expertise. However, in this RFE, caregivers are the content experts, while research consultants are the methodologists who help caregivers operationalize their ideas. Caregivers are primary investigators and first authors. As such, they learn all aspects of the research process that relate to their study. Their learning prepares them at the conclusion of their first project to move to a second and third study. As the result of an enjoyable process of learning and accomplishment, caregivers frequently want research consultants to be coauthors of a publication. The excitement over their accomplishments seems to be transferred into gratitude toward the individuals who helped them reach their goals. Consultants may or may not agree to be coauthors; the choice is theirs.

References

Bradley, H., Cantrell, D., Dollahan, K., Hall, B., Lewis, P., Merritt, S., & White, D. (2015). Evaluating preceptors: A methodological study. *Journal of Nurses Professional Development, 31*(3), 164–169. doi:10.1097/nnd.0000000000000166

Brockopp, D. Y., & Hastings-Tolsma, M. (2003). *Fundamentals of nursing research.* Sudbury, MA: Jones and Bartlett Publishers.

Brockopp, D., Downey, E., Powers, P., Vanderveer, B., Warden, S., Ryan, P., & Saleh, U. (2004). Nurses' clinical decision-making regarding the management of pain. *International Journal of Nursing Studies, 41*(631), 631–636.

Brockopp, D., Hill, K., Moe, K., & Wright, L. (2016). Transforming practice through publication: A community hospital approach to the creation of a research-intensive environment. *Journal of Nursing Administration, 46*(1), 38–42. Doi:10.1097/nna.0000000000000294

Bugajski, A., Lengerich, A., Marchese, M., Hall, B., Yackzan, S., Davies, C., & Brockopp, D. (2017). The importance of factors related to nurse retention: Using the Baptist Health Nurse Retention Questionnaire part 2. *Journal of Nursing Administration, 47*(6), 308–312. doi:10.1097/nna .0000000000000486

Groppo-Lawless S., Bugajski A., & Lengerich A. (2018). Developing and testing the diagnostic accuracy of a brief nursing dysphagia screen for pneumonia inpatients. *American Journal of Speech-Language Pathology.* In press.

Hahn, J., Byrd, R., Lengerich, A., Hench, J., Ford, C., Byrd, S., & Stoltz, R. (2015). Neonatal abstinence syndrome: The experience of infant massage. *Creative Nursing, 22*(1), 45–50. doi:10.1891 /1078-4535.22.1.45

Lewis, D. A., Sanders, L. P., & Brockopp, D. Y. (2011). The effect of three nursing interventions on thermoregulation in low birth weight infants. *Neonatal Network, 30*(3), 160–164. doi:10.1891 /0730-0832.30.3.160

Lewis, C. P., Corley, D. J., Lake, N., Brockopp, D., & Moe, K. (2015). Overcoming barriers to effective pain management: The use of professionally directed small group discussions. *Pain Management Nursing, 16*(2), 121–127. doi:10.1016/j.pmn.2014.05.002

Minnick, J. (2017). The 2017 JCR report is here! *Clarivate Analytics.* Retrieved from https://clarivate. com/blog/the-2017-jcr-release-is-here/

Schreiber, J. A., Cantrell, D., Moe, K. A., Hench, J., McKinney, E., Lewis, C., . . . , Brockopp, D. (2014). Improving knowledge, assessment, and attitudes related to pain management: evaluation of an intervention. *Pain Management Nursing, 15*(2), 474–481. doi:10.1016/j.pmn.2012.12.006

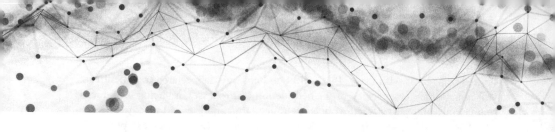

CHAPTER 8

Research-Friendly Environments: The Future

"Evidence-based practice is simply the integration of the best-possible research evidence with clinical expertise and with patient needs."

— **Malloch & Porter-O'Grady**, 2010

▶ Introduction

Given the requirements for Magnet designation, healthcare professionals' desire to improve care, and pressure on caregivers to base patient care on evidence, the importance of developing hospital environments that support and encourage research is likely to increase. As a result, traditional hospital cultures and administrative priorities may need to change. In order to prepare nurses to actively pursue evidence as a basis for practice, modifications in undergraduate nursing programs may also be necessary.

▶ Magnet Designation: Increasing Expectations

Expectations regarding nurses' involvement in research activities related to Magnet designation continue to evolve. Nurses are increasingly expected to conduct research and disseminate their findings. Asking questions, proposing solutions, and evaluating practice on a continuous basis are realistic expectations of nurses who work in a Magnet-designated setting.

At present, to maintain or achieve Magnet designation, hospital-based nurses, at a minimum, need to be comfortable reviewing patient-related data and evaluating aspects of patient care. For example, they need to understand reports that describe length of stay, patient morbidity following procedures, and inpatient falls. Interacting on a regular basis with teams that collect and analyze data related to patient care will increasingly be expected of the bedside nurse. Processes are being introduced in hospital settings that require nurses to understand, analyze, and work with data.

For example, in this research-friendly environment (RFE), the Lean process is incorporated into caregivers' daily lives. Through the introduction of Lean activities, care providers are increasingly focused on systematically improving processes of care. They use data to identify how the work gets done. They also use those data to develop and test new models of care. Nurses are learning to work with data and develop research projects based on the outcomes of those data. Newly graduated nurses could benefit from understanding this and/or other approaches that require an understanding of data.

▶ Patient Care: Changing Expectations

Most, if not all, hospital-based caregivers understand that diagnosis of illness, treatment of disease, and bedside care are continually changing. As the population in the United States ages and morbidity from chronic illness increases, changes in the complexity of patient care will also increase (McClelland & Albert, 2016). Caregivers will become aware of the continuous evolution of the healthcare environment as they personally observe patient-care issues on a daily basis. Their observations can lead them to seek assistance from individuals with expertise in research methods to design and conduct studies in order to resolve some of the problems they experience.

An expectation that caregivers must continuously work toward improving patient care can be developed within a hospital setting. As the complexity of patient care grows, there will be an increasing need to foster such an expectation. Projects and publications at this site reflect a commitment to providing optimal care within the institution.

▶ Hospital Culture: A Vision for the Future

The culture of a hospital can either support or discourage research activities initiated and conducted by caregivers. Hospital administrators' willingness to accept and support caregivers' challenges to present approaches to care is important to the development of an RFE. Comfort with change is an important characteristic of an environment that encourages research. A supportive culture encourages questioning, acknowledges success, and provides adequate resources. Proactive leadership is essential in developing an RFE.

Encouraging questioning of present practices usually begins at the unit level within a hospital. Caregivers at the bedside who feel comfortable reporting patient-care concerns or suggesting alternative approaches to care to their managers are likely to become involved in projects that might change practice. Leaders at all levels who welcome criticism of present practices regarding patient care are, directly or indirectly, developing an environment that supports research activities.

As acuity levels continue to rise in hospital settings, caregivers' responsibilities will increase. For any number of reasons, recognition of caregivers' efforts at the bedside is warranted. Acknowledgment of work well done in research activities is important and can take many forms. In relation to research, email messages to all employees announcing successes and newsletters that include descriptions of studies can acknowledge caregiver efforts. Personal interactions between administrators and caregivers that encourage and support research activities can also motivate staff to continue to develop and conduct studies. A symposium for caregivers to present their research, held annually, can also support and encourage caregivers to engage in research activities.

For nurses, including research activities on a clinical ladder is another strategy that can foster interest in research. In this RFE, nurses on the clinical ladder often begin their research requirement by conducting a critical appraisal of the literature. This appraisal consists of using bullet points to describe the major issues found in five or six recent data-based articles in an area of their interest. At the conclusion of the appraisal, nurses make recommendations related to practice based on their reading, resulting in points supporting their advancement on the ladder. Following this activity, they frequently move to other components of the research process within the same area of interest.

▶ Attitudes Toward Research: A New Direction

Positive attitudes toward caregivers conducting research are a necessary component of the development and maintenance of an RFE. Unfortunately, in nursing, tradition has held that graduate degrees are required in order to conduct research. Specifically, baccalaureate-prepared nurses are expected only to evaluate research findings, apply them to patient situations, and assist in one component of the research process—that is, the development of a research question (Hedges & Williams, 2014). This position has led faculty in nursing programs to design research courses that do not teach students the steps necessary to conduct research. In addition, a lack of knowledge of the research process and resistance to nurses at the bedside acting as principal investigators are not uncommon (Stutzman et al., 2016).

A recommendation resulting from the experience in this RFE would be to add an additional expectation of baccalaureate and associate-degree nurses to conduct research with assistance. Baccalaureate-prepared nurses as well as associate-degree nurses can, with appropriate mentoring, design and conduct studies and publish their findings.

In this RFE, two experienced nurses prepared at the associate-degree level have conducted studies and published their findings in peer-reviewed journals (Hahn et al., 2015; Thompson, Moe, & Lewis, 2014). In addition to disseminating their findings to other institutions through publication, most importantly their results impacted practice within this RFE. The knowledge of experienced caregivers regarding patient care is extensive and invaluable (Stutzman et al., 2016). The recommendation throughout this text is to help caregivers translate that knowledge into meaningful changes in patient care through designing and conducting studies.

▶ Use of Resources: A Recommendation for the Future

How resources, such as the institutional review board (IRB), library, and research office, are constructed and used is another factor to consider when developing an RFE.

There is a difference between IRBs that see their task as doing everything possible to help caregivers conduct research and those IRBs that are more concerned about the details of an application than helping new investigators meet their goals. In addition, it has been suggested that IRBs that include nurses as members are more likely to approve research proposals submitted by nurses (Stutzman et al., 2016). Similarly, librarians who understand the responsibilities of caregivers and are willing to provide whatever help they need to reach their goals fosters an ongoing interest in the research process. Most important is the need for research consultants who are excited about mentoring caregivers, teaching them to develop research skills, and working side by side with principal investigators as they write for publication.

There are a number of approaches presently used to support hospital-based, caregiver-initiated research. In some hospital settings, individuals are hired to assist caregivers to conduct research in addition to developing and maintaining their own research program (Albert, 2016). While this approach ensures the maintenance of consultants' research skills, the focus of their activities may be deflected from that of supporting caregivers' initiatives.

In medical centers associated with universities, faculty members from nursing and allied health often conduct research within the hospital setting. A combination of these approaches exists in this RFE. Faculty from universities are welcome to conduct research that is in keeping with hospital goals, and research consultants may design and conduct studies. However, consultants' primary responsibility is to assist other caregivers to engage in research. No pressure is exerted on consultants to maintain a program of research.

Within this RFE, consultants can be compared to clinical experts. For example, pain team members, who provide assistance to caregivers related to managing their patients' pain, perform in a similar fashion to research consultants. Ongoing assistance is provided, and, as learning takes place, less assistance is needed. As an example, one of the nurses prepared at the associate-degree level who published her work on neonatal abstinence syndrome (NAS) babies is preparing to conduct a second, funded study.

▶ Administration: A Different Kind

If the future of hospitals includes caregiver-initiated research, administrators may need to modify their traditional roles. Given the number of nurses who work in a hospital setting, chief nursing officers (CNOs), in particular, can contribute greatly to the development of an environment that supports and encourages research. Given that many CNOs are not recent or current students, they may need to connect with area nursing programs in order to understand nursing students' preparation related to research. Understanding nursing curricula can help CNOs design experiences for new employees that will help them transition successfully from education to practice.

CNOs and senior nurse leaders need to understand what new graduates have learned regarding the research process as well as their comfort level regarding research. Questions such as "Do they understand the issue of human subjects' protection?" or "Have they had any experience designing studies or have they focused solely on searching the literature?" or "Do they understand Magnet designation and what it means in relation to research and the bedside provider?" need to be addressed. This kind of information can influence residency programs as well as initial orientation programs.

While senior administration may support and encourage research activities throughout a hospital, unless administrators at the unit level are equally supportive, little research activity is likely to occur. Leaders at all levels will need to support, encourage, and participate in healthcare professionals' efforts to improve patient care through conducting research. Managers at the unit level may be the first individuals to hear about a caregiver's desire to design a study.

Unit leaders, particularly those who are new to the position, may not have the knowledge and skills to support their staff who are conducting research. These individuals are instrumental in setting the tone for engagement and inclusion of staff on a unit. In many organizations, nursing leaders have been long-term staff members and may have graduated from nursing programs prior to the inclusion of a research course in the curriculum.

Research consultants, librarians, and IRB coordinators will need to assist these individuals to gain the skills necessary to support their staff as they become involved in research activities. Classes can be held or individual discussions can be scheduled. Developing an awareness of resources available for unit leaders as well as their staff is an important step in assisting managers to feel comfortable supporting their staff in research activities. Encouraging managers to attend an annual symposium where they can learn what caregivers are doing in terms of research can also help them to support research activities.

Leaders can develop residency programs for nurses as they transition from school to practice that include information regarding the importance of research activities as they embark on their careers. During residency programs, presenters can attempt to modify negative attitudes toward research, describe the importance of research within a Magnet-designated setting, and describe the resources that are available to them. Basic research principles, IRB requirements, and the importance of improving practice through evidence can also be presented.

CNOs can develop relationships within the academic community that can foster the development of an RFE. This RFE has become known as a laboratory for caregiver-initiated research. As long as a study is in agreement with the hospital's mission, purpose, and goals, a proposed study will be reviewed. When faculty of nearby colleges conduct research in an RFE, positive outcomes for the hospital can include improvements in patient care, inclusion of caregivers in the research process (including publication), and role modeling of research activities for staff. In addition, faculty may experience practice changes that can influence curriculum development within their colleges. An associate professor and experienced researcher from a local university are presently conducting a study in this RFE (see **BOX 8-1**).

On occasion, individuals with expertise in a particular area are invited to conduct research at the hospital. These individuals work together with research consultants as needed. For example, a nursing faculty member from a local university, internationally recognized for her work with nurse manager span of control and professional support, was asked to conduct a project at this RFE. When the CNO decided to review the current curriculum of the hospital's Evolving Leaders program, an internal leadership development program, she commissioned this professor to conduct a study to identify up-to-date content and evaluation processes. Research consultants supported the project as needed.

> ### 👥 BOX 8-1 Kristin Ashford, RN, MSN, PhD, FAAN: E-cigarettes and Pregnancy
>
> Kristin Ashford, Associate Professor at a local university, is conducting a study to examine the health effects of e-cigarettes on pregnant women and their babies. Tobacco use during pregnancy is the most modifiable risk associated with adverse birth outcome, yet nearly one in four women in this state continue to use tobacco products during pregnancy. E-cigarettes also contain varied (unregulated) concentrations of nicotine.
>
> Her goal is to determine the effects of e-cigarettes (and dual use, cigarettes plus e-cigarettes) on perinatal biomarkers and birth outcomes. Three hundred sixty pregnant women will be recruited. Participants will complete a survey to measure tobacco-related behaviors and provide perinatal biomarkers at four time points (each trimester and postpartum). Data analysis will include a series of repeated analyses of covariance (ANCOVAs) to determine the association of perinatal cigarette smoking (conventional, e-cigarettes only, and dual use) with perinatal biomarkers. A one-way ANCOVA will be used to determine the association with birth outcomes. Primary biomarker measures include expired air carbon monoxide, urine and serum cotinine, serum immune markers, and urinary NNAL. Gestational age at birth and birthweight are the primary birth outcomes.
>
> Until more data about the effects of e-cigarettes and dual use on perinatal immune response and birth outcomes are available, promotion of e-cigarettes during pregnancy would be premature. There is an urgent need to investigate the impact of e-cigarettes and dual use on perinatal biomarkers and birth outcomes. The lack of research may unnecessarily place women—and their babies—at risk for lifelong adverse health outcomes.

Working together with faculty from local universities on research activities fosters valuable relationships that can benefit healthcare providers throughout the institution. Short-term engagements of this kind move the hospital forward and contribute to the maintenance of an RFE. These engagements also model a behavior of studying issues carefully before making change. For example, the CNO identified a need to work with a medical-surgical unit in an effort to improve engagement and retention of staff. She asked a nursing faculty member at a nearby university who had extensive experience with appreciative inquiry and many years of nursing leadership to design a project that might improve both engagement and retention. The unit in question had been through major changes. A new manager was put in place at the same time that the unit moved to a different location. The research project is described in **BOX 8-2**.

Hospital administrators are often concerned regarding the cost of a new program. Over the years, conversations with administrators from other hospitals have revealed misperceptions regarding the cost of developing an environment that encourages research. There is some concern that creating an office dedicated to supporting research activities would be resource intensive. In reality, RFEs can be cost conservative, centered on part-time expertise and PhD student affiliations. Even so, the CNO may need to develop a business case relating clinical benefits of findings to further justify research office staffing.

> ### 👥 BOX 8-2 Karen Stefaniak, RN, PhD: Staff Nurses and Appreciative Inquiry
>
> This project was designed to include both qualitative and quantitative methods. Working with a hospital administrator and Karen, consultants developed a questionnaire to assess nurses' perceptions of the current work environment. Following approval by IRB, staff on the unit who were willing to participate completed the questionnaire. Appreciative inquiry is the strategy used to identify those components of the workplace that are "appreciated" or positive. Appreciative inquiry provided the framework for conducting focus groups. Three staff nurses were co-investigators on the project. They reviewed and edited the focus group discussion guide and recorded discussions. As a result of both responses to the questionnaire and group discussions, organizational practices that could be modified to improve engagement and retention included bedside hand-off, shift huddles, management team feedback to staff, and the shared governance council. The staff nurse co-investigators are currently leading staff nurse teams to address identified issues incorporating appreciative inquiry into their approach.

▶ The Profession of Nursing: Future Directions

In order to engage hospital-based caregivers in research activities, the nursing profession may need to consider "research" as a set of skills that can be learned in the clinical setting and applied in specific situations. There has been a tendency to categorize nurses, based on degree obtained, in terms of whether or not they can conduct research. A present example is related to the clinical doctorate in nursing (DNP). Nurses holding clinical doctorates are frequently directed to conduct quality improvement projects but not research projects (Nelson, Cook, & Raterink, 2013). As previously mentioned baccalaureate- or associate degree–prepared nurses are not thought capable of initiating and directing studies.

The recommendation for the future, based on the experience in this RFE, is to judge capability for conducting research on the individual and not on a particular degree obtained. Based on prior research experience, varying degrees of assistance may be necessary to enable caregivers to conduct research. The value of caregivers' clinical experience is such that providing assistance to them in order to test their ideas is worth the expenditure of resources.

▶ Developing a Research-Friendly Environment: Hospital-Based Strategies

There are a number of strategies presently in place that can assist in the development of an environment that supports and encourages research. **TABLE 8-1** outlines these strategies, which are discussed below.

TABLE 8-1 Strategies to Assist in the Development of an RFE				
Strategy	**Goal**	**Required Resources**	**Outcomes**	**Reference**
The Neuroscience Nursing Center Research Fellowship	To engage nurses at all levels of clinical practice in research activities	Director, program manager, scientific writer, grants/contracts manager, ad hoc affiliations with faculty content experts *University affiliated*	In approximately 1 year, training provided for 150 nurses; 20 abstract/posters accepted at regional (2), national (6), and international (4) conferences; 11 manuscripts submitted for publication: 7 accepted, 7 under review	Stutzman et al., 2016
Nursing Fellowship Program	To expand the potential of nurses to conduct research	Professor emeritus *Hospital based*	One participant was awarded a grant ($13,000), one fellow's work may result in a practice change, one fellow's work will be used by marketing to develop health education materials	Mason, Lambton, & Fernandes, 2017
Research Training Program for Point-of-Care Clinicians	To support nurses in conducting small-scale research projects	Research leader, advisory committee, experienced researchers/mentors *University affiliated*	Seven publications in peer-reviewed journals, 28 presentations at national or international conferences	Black, Bungay, Mackay, Balneaves, & Garossino, 2016; Black, Balneaves, Garossino, Puyat, & Qian, 2015

Strategy	Goal	Required Resources	Outcomes	Reference
The Research Consultation Model	To assist hospital-based caregivers to conduct research	Two PhD-prepared, part-time (20 hrs/week) consultants, one PhD student in nursing or psychology *Hospital based*	Between 2013 and 2017, 36 publications in peer-reviewed journals and $50,122 in funding received	Brockopp, Moe, Corley, & Schreiber, 2013; Brockopp, Hill, Moe, & Wright, 2016

The Neuroscience Nursing Research Center Fellowship Model

This model was developed at a university-associated hospital to involve nurses at all levels of practice to engage in research activities (Stutzman et al., 2016). The following four pathways exist in this model: research fellowships, student-nurse internships, didactic training, and research consultation. At the time of publication, 150 nurses had received research training.

Requirements for Participation

Nurses at the bedside are the focus of the program. In order to participate in this training program, they are required to submit an application. They prepare a brief description of their topic of interest and obtain two letters of recommendation. Their nurse manager must support their participation in the program.

Program Activities

Following selection, fellows in this model complete online training modules related to research and begin to construct a research protocol. Approximately 2 months after acceptance as a fellow, participants experience an 8-hour "boot camp." They are expected, as fellows, to complete a study as primary investigator and submit findings for publication. Time expected for fellows to complete their work is approximately 18 months.

Resources Required

Individuals with expertise in grant writing and statistics participate in this model. In addition, an individual with management skills, research coordinators, medical and nursing interns, and faculty participants assist fellows to meet their goals. An advisory board also plays a role in this model. Five individuals representing the medical and academic community constitute a board that meets annually. This board addresses issues related to nursing research, cost of program, and overall management of activities.

Outcomes of the Neuroscience Nursing Research Center Model

Publication of research findings and/or presentations at national and international conferences are desired outcomes of this model. In addition to publications and presentations, it appears that multiple individuals are learning the value of research as well as skills necessary to conduct research. Given the setting, a hospital associated with a university, research expertise is more readily available than in many community hospital environments.

The Nursing Fellowship Program

This program includes nurses and allied health professionals who provide care at the bedside (Mason, Lambton, & Fernandez, 2017). The goal of this fellowship program is to provide the skills needed for caregivers at the bedside to conduct independent research. This program is 1 year in length and provides release time (12 hours) from work. Fellows are expected to give an oral presentation and submit a grant proposal (internal or external).

Requirements for Participation

In order to apply, caregivers must have completed 1 year of employment, their topic of interest needs to fit with program goals, and proposed research must be designed so that completion in 1 year is possible. Candidates complete an application that describes their interests and accomplishments. They must also include a letter of support from their managers.

Program Activities

Participants in this program meet once a month in a formal classroom setting. They study research topics such as research ethics, protocol development, statistics, grant writing, and manuscript writing. In addition to formal classroom work, they meet with individuals who have expertise related to IRB, grant writing, and statistical analysis.

Resources Required

A professor emeritus developed the curriculum for this fellowship. She taught each class and was available for individual meetings. Additional assistance was available in relation to research methods. An evaluation of this program revealed a greater need for support of participants than planned. In addition, fellows had difficulty meeting each of the monthly scheduled classes. Recommendations for future programs included scheduling 10 rather than 12 classes, providing additional independent support, and modifying the curriculum.

Outcomes of the Nursing Fellowship Program

Outcomes of this program included funding of a grant proposal, building a foundation for future research, and considering possible changes in practice. Fellows write letters of inquiry to journal editors regarding their projects; however, acceptances are not reported.

Research Training Program for Point-of-Care Clinicians

The goal of this program is to enable nurses at the bedside to conduct small research projects that could lead to practice change (Black, Bungay, Mackay, Balneaves, & Garossino, 2016; Black, Balneaves, Garossino, Puyat, & Qian, 2015). Upon completion of the program, nurse graduates would be able to identify evidence needed to change practice, integrate evidence into practice, and develop strategies that would enable them to discover the knowledge necessary to address patient-care problems. The focus of this program is on mentorship. Mentors are viewed as an essential component of the learning process in relation to research skills.

Requirements for Participation

Teams of individuals wanting to conduct research apply to receive this training. Each team is required to have one member practicing at the bedside who has no other responsibilities, such as research or administration. Teams submit letters of intent that describe membership of the team as well as the idea the team wants to study. Feasibility of conducting the study and the potential for meaningful outcomes are criteria for acceptance. Once teams are accepted, they write a research proposal. Based on the quality of proposals, teams may receive funding ranging from $2,000 to $5,000 to support their work.

Program Activities

Research teams approved for training in this program attend three workshops. These workshops focus on research methods, ethics, and strategies for searching the literature. Working with an assigned mentor, teams are given 3 months following the workshops to develop a brief proposal. Proposals are evaluated using criteria of feasibility, sound research design, and potential outcomes. Teams who meet these criteria receive funding for their studies. They conduct their studies over a 1-year period.

Resources Required

Experienced researchers, a research leader, and an advisory committee are the resources dedicated to this program. Each team has an experienced researcher who mentors them throughout their study. A research leader organizes the program, seeks external funding, and organizes workshops to assist teams to publish their findings. The advisory committee, which includes clinicians and faculty, provides oversight for the program.

The Research Consultation Model

The Research Consultation Model is the approach described in this text (Brockopp, Moe, Corley, & Schreiber, 2013; Brockopp, Hill, Moe, & Wright, 2016). This model is designed to enable caregivers from nursing, medicine, and allied health to conduct research and publish their findings. Feasibility, congruence with hospital mission and goals, and potential to improve practice are criteria used to evaluate ideas proposed by caregivers. Although classes may be held as requested, the major focus of this model is on interpersonal relationships that involve mentoring, coaching, and teaching.

A similar model exists at the Cleveland Clinic (Albert, 2016), although it is designed to engage only nurses in research.

Requirements for Participation

All caregivers employed at the institution are eligible for participation in this model. In addition, students not employed by the institution, from local or regional universities, may also avail themselves of consultants' expertise. Permission to work with nonemployees is given by the CNO based on the match of the topic of interest with hospital goals and mission. Neither degree held nor professional affiliation is a criterion for consideration when caregivers approach consultants for assistance with research.

Program Activities

This model is characterized by meetings between research consultants and caregivers, on a regular basis, as projects are designed, studies are conducted, and findings are submitted for publication. Relationships are established that enable caregivers to learn from individuals whose goal is to help them to be as successful as possible in meeting their goals.

Resources Required

In this model, individuals with research expertise are required to teach and mentor caregivers interested in conducting research. PhD-prepared researchers and PhD students in nursing and psychology fill this role. Two part-time researchers and one part-time PhD student presently support caregivers. Expertise in designing and conducting research, analyzing data, and writing for publication is essential.

Outcomes of the Research Consultation Model

Publishing findings in peer-reviewed journals is a major goal of this model. During the years 2013 to 2017, an average of 7.2 acceptances per year of manuscripts occurred. Approximately 40 projects are ongoing at any point in time.

Developing a Research-Friendly Environment: Hospital-Based Strategies: Summary

Similarities in the above strategies used to engage hospital-based caregivers in research are the rationale for developing research-intensive opportunities, desired outcomes, and expertise involved. Differences include participant identification, formality of offering, expectations, and teaching/learning methods.

Participant Identification: Differences

Three of the strategies are focused on nurses; one includes all hospital-based caregivers. The focus on nurses is related to their numbers in a hospital setting, their continuous relationships with patients, and their education in problem solving. Nurses constitute the largest number of healthcare providers in hospitals. Through their continuous contact with patients, they are best able to identify present and potential problems related to patient care. Magnet designation has played a major role in encouraging nurses to be actively involved in research. One strategy, the Research Consultation Model, provides training for all interested healthcare professionals. An advantage of this model is the likelihood that interprofessional projects will occur.

Formality of Offerings: Differences

The Research Consultation Model is an informal strategy that provides teaching and mentoring on an "as come" basis. There are no applications and no required timelines for completion of activities. The other strategies are time limited and have several requirements for participants to engage in classes, workshops, or assigned mentoring relationships. While the lack of formality allows caregivers to work at their own pace, a more formal situation is less likely to result in procrastination when busy professionals are involved.

Expectations: Differences

In each of the fellowships, there is a completion date for specified tasks. Proposals, manuscripts, and/or presentations may be required. Failure to graduate from the program is a consequence of not completing required tasks. Consultants working with the Research Consultation Model expect that caregivers will continue to work with them until completion of their projects; however, there is no consequence for not completing their work. In this model, publication of findings is an expectation. Given few resources for travel, presentation at regional or national conferences is not emphasized.

Teaching/Learning Methods: Differences

Lecturing in formal classes or workshop settings is characteristic of the fellowships offered. Didactic content is presented prior to participants' engaging in the research process. Experts in research methods, statistics, and writing for publication provide content for coursework. In the Research Consultation Model, learning takes place as caregivers conduct their studies. One-on-one relationships are developed between consultants and caregivers that remain from the initiation of a project to submitting a manuscript for publication.

Rationale for Strategies: Similarities

The rationale given for the development of each strategy is similar. The need to base practice on evidence, the view of nurses as a particularly appropriate group of caregivers to include in research activities, and a desire for hospitals to gain Magnet designation were given as reasons for offering opportunities for caregivers to conduct research.

Desired Outcomes: Similarities

Learning research skills, developing and conducting a study, and disseminating findings were expected in each strategy described. While the emphasis on each outcome as well as methods to reach each outcome differed, desired outcomes were similar. Overall, strategies were designed to assist caregivers to obtain evidence to support practice on a continuous basis by conducting research.

Expertise Involved: Similarities

Although individual backgrounds might differ, the expertise required is similar for each strategy. Knowledge of research methods and expertise in statistical analysis, grant writing, and writing for publication was available in each program. In some instances, one individual provided training in all areas; in others, experts in each area contributed to the program.

Selecting strategies to engage hospital-based caregivers in research may vary depending on a number of factors. The work environment in terms of acceptance of change, theoretical underpinnings for practice, availability of research expertise, desire for Magnet designation, and a goal of providing patient care based on evidence may influence decisions. Fellowships may be appropriate in a university medical center, while providing research consultation may be more effective in a community hospital. At this point in time, it appears that hospitals are filling a gap in the incoming knowledge of caregivers as they graduate from their educational programs.

▶ Caregiver Education: Future Strategies and Recommendations

A number of questions remain regarding the role played by education in preparing individuals to practice in hospital settings. For example, why do hospitals need to provide additional education for caregivers in relation to basic research skills? Are nurses specifically, as reported in 2008 (Ravert & Merrill, 2008), practicing more on the basis of tradition rather than evidence? Is the nursing profession focused more on categorizing research skill levels in terms of specific degrees rather than clinical ability and healthcare needs? If the answer to these questions is in the affirmative, changes in education are needed.

In the future, an understanding of evidence in terms of generation of knowledge as well as clinical application is likely to be essential for individuals providing care at the bedside. Recent literature speaks to the need for caregivers to ask questions relative to patient care and seek means of resolving patient-care problems through research. Barriers are present, however, in both hospital and university settings. Nurses, in particular, lack training to conduct research, are not viewed as competent principal investigators, and frequently do not have access to mentors (Stutzman et al., 2016).

There is some agreement that nursing education needs to change. Additional skills are required if nurses are to care for patients in an environment that embraces evidence-based practice. Teaching methods and traditional ways of thinking may need to be modified. The value of research can be conveyed in every course rather than limited to one three-credit offering. Given that, for most students, learning related to clinical issues and skills is their major priority, they often view the research course as something they have to contend with and then forget. If the need for evidence as it relates to practice was threaded throughout the curriculum, the value of research would be clear (Malloch & O'Grady, 2010).

Overall curriculum change that integrates the generation of evidence into each course is one possible modification of present nursing curricula. Another possibility is to change courses in research to focus on clinical issues of interest. These courses could also involve students in learning how to conduct research rather than focusing solely on reviewing the literature.

Providing a research course that will engage students in the process of designing and conducting studies is another strategy that may enable new graduates to actively participate in hospital-based research activities. A possible course syllabus is provided in **TABLE 8-2**.

TABLE 8-2 Course Title: Transforming Practice Through Research				
Goal	**Description**	**Learning Outcomes**	**Teaching/ Learning Methods**	**Evaluation**
The goals of this course are to engage students in the conduct of research by teaching basic research skills and to convey the value of evidence as a foundation for clinical practice.	Students, based on a topic of clinical interest, must select and critically appraise five data-based articles related to their topic. Then, in groups of two to five, they must use the research process to write a study proposal on the same topic.	After completion of the course, students will be able to describe major categories of research (quantitative/ qualitative), describe experimental versus non-experimental research designs, write research questions, critically appraise five data-based articles related to a specific clinical topic, apply each of the steps in the research process, write a research proposal following specified headings, and analyze ethical issues related to their proposed study.	Brief lectures and small group discussions. Occasional talks by hospital-based researchers on their studies.	Group proposals completed at the end of the semester submitted in writing and presented to the class (75%). Individual critical appraisals of the literature submitted at mid-term (25%).

A course that takes students through each step of the research process can prepare them to be actively involved in research activities in the hospital setting. Students who have had clinical experiences in their educational programs can readily identify patient-care issues. With assistance, they can translate these issues into a research question and, from there, address each step in the research process. They learn each step within the framework of their area of interest, preparing them to develop a study proposal.

In addition to modifying a nursing curriculum or offering a different kind of research course, there are strategies that colleges can offer to enhance students' interest in research and better prepare them to engage in research activities in a hospital setting. A Nurse Scholars elective course and providing research internships are two strategies that can engage undergraduate students in research. **TABLE 8-3** outlines these strategies.

The Nurse Scholars Strategy

A Nurse Scholars option for undergraduate students permits them to examine areas of clinical interest in depth. Students can suggest speakers with particular expertise and/or investigate a specific area on their own and present to class. Classroom time enables them to understand how to examine a topic of interest and how to access and analyze the evidence available related to that topic.

Participant Requirements

Students who apply to be Nurse Scholars are generally those individuals who have extra time and are academically successful. They frequently have graduate school in mind and want to prepare themselves for advanced work. An option for a program is to require a specific Grade Point Average (GPA) in order to join Nurse Scholars. Another option is to interview applicants and verify their ability to commit to the time required as well as their ability to engage in expected activities.

Activities

Students are expected to prepare for discussions of specific topics at each meeting of Scholars. In addition, they discuss their plans for constructing a project. All projects are based on the evidence underlying the topic of interest. For example, there is evidence to suggest that breastfeeding can lead to positive outcomes for mothers and babies. A student might design a brochure to be distributed at a public health clinic encouraging women to breastfeed. The brochure would be based on available evidence. Another student might investigate issues related to wound care among the elderly. A PowerPoint presentation regarding nurse assessment of skin breakdown would be an acceptable project.

Potential Outcomes

Anecdotal information from 5 years of guiding a Nurse Scholars program suggests that these students learn a great deal regarding how to access and use evidence. They also begin to understand the value of evidence when providing patient care. On a practical note, approximately 20% of scholars each year applied to graduate school at completion of their program of study. They included their experience as a Nurse

TABLE 8-3 Strategies to Engage Undergraduate Nursing Students in Research			
Strategy	**Participant Requirements**	**Activities**	**Outcomes**
Nurse Scholars (1 to 3 credit elective course) Suggested class size: 12 to 15	A grade point average (GPA) can be set if desirable. Offered to sophomores, juniors, and seniors if curriculum permits.	Weekly discussions (depending on credit hours, 1- to 3-hour meetings) Project required	Letter grade based on participation in discussions and final project or Pass/Fail. Students may choose either approach. "Enhanced learning related to the value of research project" can be included on resume.
Nursing research internship (1 to 3 credit independent study elective course: 1 credit = 4 hours of research practicum)	A GPA can be set if desirable. Offered to sophomores, juniors, and seniors depending on placement of research course and if curriculum permits.	Based on student interest, advisor assists the student to identify a research mentor (either faculty or a researcher at a local hospital). Advisor and student meet with the mentor to discuss research activities that will occur throughout the semester. Expected outcomes are negotiated.	Letter grade based on ongoing research activities and meeting expected outcome. or Pass/Fail. Students may choose either approach. Depending on number of semesters chosen by students, they may be included in abstracts submitted for presentation or manuscripts submitted for publication.

Scholar on their applications and felt confident that this inclusion would benefit them in terms of acceptance.

The Nurse Research Internship

The internship model is one that provides nursing students with actual experience with the research process. In order to offer an internship, a number of researchers, either faculty or hospital based, need to be available to mentor students. In the best-case scenario, students are able to find a mentor whose research is of interest to them. For the most in-depth experience, students could participate in an internship experience for three semesters; if they intern for more than one semester, they have a better chance of participating in the entire study process.

Participant Requirements

The internship experience can be open to all students, or students can be selected in terms of a specific GPA or interview. Time available can be a major factor that limits students' involvement given the clinical experiences already embedded within nursing curricula. To be successful, students must spend 4 hours a week with their mentor and meet with their advisor as needed.

Activities

Interns may be involved in any part of the research process. It is the responsibility of the mentor to ensure that, regardless of the component of the research process that students are working on, they need to understand all aspects of the study. They may join a mentor at the beginning of a study and assist with research design. Students participate in working with many members of the mentor's team. For example, research intern students who complete IRB and human subjects training can assist their mentor's team in the clinical setting. In this RFE, research intern students are paired with nurses conducting research a few times throughout the semester. They may also assist with data entry, data analysis, and/or writing a manuscript.

Potential Outcomes

Students have hands-on experience as research interns. They learn about the research process and also gain an in-depth understanding of some of the difficulties encountered when conducting studies. Depending on their mentors, interns may also attend monthly research meetings and local, regional, or national conferences and be listed as a copresenter. They may also be included as a coauthor on a publication. Presentation and publication opportunities are usually only available to those interns who spend more than one semester as an intern.

Unfortunately, both Nurse Scholars and research internships can only be offered to a select group of students. Even so, such opportunities can move a college environment toward one that emphasizes the importance of seeking evidence for practice and conducting research.

▶ Chapter Summary

This chapter focused on the need to develop environments within hospitals that support caregiver-initiated research. Necessary resources were identified and strategies for both hospital and educational settings were described. Expertise was addressed in terms of content needed as well as attitudes of consultants that help to move caregivers toward their research goals.

Hospital-based strategies include nurse fellowships, research training programs, and the provision of individual research consultation. The goals for each strategy are the same. Encouraging and supporting caregivers to conduct research given appropriate assistance is embedded in each strategy. Strategies aimed toward the educational preparation of nurses relative to research include limited offerings for undergraduate students such as Nurse Scholars programs and research internships. In addition, threading research and the need for evidence to support practice throughout the curriculum and modifying research courses to include basic steps in the research process are suggested.

A possible gap between hospital needs and educational offerings is identified. Particularly in nursing, it seems that barriers to nurses at the bedside actively participating in research remain. In this profession, it appears that an emphasis on degree obtained, rather than the ability of a given caregiver, is a barrier to bedside nurses' actively participating in research. In addition, the tendency of undergraduate research courses to focus on reviewing literature rather than learning the steps involved in conducting research can prevent nurses from active involvement in designing and conducting studies.

Recent publications on the topic of strategies designed to increase hospital-based nurse involvement in research (Black et al., 2015; Black et al., 2016; Mason, Lambton, & Fernandes, 2017; Stutzman et al., 2016) suggest that attitudes and activities are evolving. The movement appears to be in the direction of developing and maintaining hospital environments that encourage and support caregiver-initiated research.

References

Albert, N. (2016). *Building and sustaining a hospital-based nursing research program*. New York, NY: Springer.

Black, A., Bungay, V., Mackay, M., Balneaves, L., & Garossino, C. (2016). Understanding mentorship in a research training program for point-of-care clinicians. *Journal of Nursing Administration, 46*(9), 444–448.

Black, A., Balneaves, L., Garossino, C., Puyat, J., & Qian, H. (2015). Promoting evidence-based practice through a research training program for point-of-care clinicians. *Journal of Nursing Administration, 45*(1), 14–20.

Brockopp, D., Moe, K., Corley, D., & Schreiber, J. (2013). The Baptist Health Lexington evidence-based practice model: A five-year journey. *Journal of Nursing Administration, 43*(4), 187–193.

Brockopp, D., Hill, K., Moe, K., & Wright, L. (2016). Transforming practice through publication: A community hospital approach to the creation of a research-intensive environment. *Journal of Administration, 46*(1), 38–42. doi:10.1097/nna.0000000000000294

Hahn, J., Byrd, R., Lengerich, A., Hench, J., Ford, C., Byrd, S., & Stoltz, R. (2015). Neonatal abstinence syndrome: The experience of infant massage. *Creative Nursing, 22*(1), 45–50. doi:10.1891/1078-4535.22.1.45

Hedges, C., & Williams, B. (2014). *Anatomy of research for nurses*. Indianapolis, IN: Sigma Theta Tau International.

Mason, B., Lambton, J., & Fernandes, R. (2017). Supporting clinical nurses through a research fellowship. *Journal of Nursing Administration, 47*(11), 529–531.

McClelland, N., & Albert, N. (2016). Creating a vision for nursing research by understanding benefits. In N. Albert (Ed.), *Building and sustaining a hospital-based nursing research program*. New York, NY: Springer: 1-11.

Thompson, M., Moe, K., & Lewis, C. P. (2014). The effects of music on diminishing anxiety among preoperative patients. *Journal of Radiology Nursing, 33*(4), 199–202.

Watson, J. (1985). *Nursing: The philosophy and science of caring*. Boulder, CO: University Press of Colorado.

Stutzman, S., Olson, D., Supnet, C., Harper, C., Brown-Clere, S., McCulley, B., & Goldberg, M. (2016). Promoting bedside nurse-led research through a dedicated neuroscience nursing research fellowship. *Journal of Nursing Administration, 46*(12), 648–653.

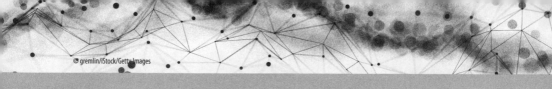

Index

Note: Page numbers followed by "*b*" denote boxes, "*f*" denote figures, and "*t*" denote tables.

A

abstracts, 151–153, 152*t*, 153*b*
ACA. *See* Patient Protection and Affordable Care Act
acute care setting, research-friendly environment in
  evidence-based practice
    achieving, 6–9
    benefits and barriers, 2–3, 2*b*
    defined, 7
    gathering evidence, 9
    methods. *See* evidence-based practice (EBP), methods
    healthcare system, 4
    Magnet designation, 4–5
    nursing practice, 5–6
administration, future of, 172–174, 174–175*b*
adult learning, 34
American Nurses Credentialing Center (ANCC), 4
analysis of covariance (ANCOVA), 137
analysis of variance (ANOVA), 136–137, 137–138*b*
analysis phase, Research-Friendly Environment Model
  content analysis, 58, 59*b*
  descriptive statistical analysis, 59, 59*b*
  inferential statistical analysis, 59–61
ANCC. *See* American Nurses Credentialing Center
ANCOVA. *See* analysis of covariance
ANOVA. *See* analysis of variance
application phase, Research-Friendly Environment Model, 56–57
  institutional review board approval, 57
Ashford, Kristin, 174*b*
association. *See* relationship
authors, response to, 166
authorship, 155

B

Baptist Health High Risk Falls Assessment (BHHRFA), 9, 48, 83
  frequency table of total scores for, 143–144*t*
  histogram for total scores for, 145*f*
Baptist Health Lexington Grid, 27, 28–29*t*, 70*t*
Baptist Health Nurse Retention Questionnaire (BHNRQ), 52*b*, 84*b*, 110*b*, 113*b*, 137*b*
BHHRFA. *See* Baptist Health High Risk Falls Assessment
BHNRQ. *See* Baptist Health Nurse Retention Questionnaire
biases, 89
Bonferroni correction, 135, 136, 136*b*
Bowles, Lindsay, 49*b*, 158*b*
Bradley, Heather, 111*b*
Bragg, Linda, 35*b*
Brockopp Warden Pain Knowledge Questionnaire, 110
Bugajski, Drew, 52*b*, 84*b*, 137*b*, 145*b*

C

cardiac rehabilitation, effect of music on, 49*b*
caregiver education, 182–184, 183*t*, 184*t*
  Nurse Research Internship, 185–186
  Nurse Scholars Strategy, 184–185
caregivers
  defined, 45
  procedures used by, 54
case studies, 84, 84*b*
Catheter Associated Urinary Tract Infections (CAUTIs), 45
CAUTIs. *See* Catheter Associated Urinary Tract Infections
chi-square analysis, 139, 140*t*

chief nursing officers (CNOs), 24, 27
  future, 172–173
  generous leadership activities, 30–33, 32*b*
closed-ended items, 105, 105–106*b*
CNOs. *See* chief nursing officers
coauthorship, 147, 155, 155*b*
collaborative writing, 160–161, 162*b*
compliance, 117
computer software, 124
conceptual frameworks, 25–26
confidence intervals, 130, 130*b*
consistency over time, 114–115, 115*b*
  internal consistency, 115
  interrater reliability, 115, 116*b*
  parallel form equivalence, 115
consistent temperature protocol, 54
construct validity, 111–112, 113*b*
content analysis, 58, 59*b*
content validity, 109–111, 110–111*b*
content validity index (CVI), 110, 111*b*
convenience sample, 87
Corley, Donna, 114*b*
correlational designs, 84–85
correlational statistical tests, 133–134, 134*b*
cover letter, 117–118
criterion-referenced measures, 96
criterion-related validity, 112–113

D

DASS. *See* Distress Anxiety Stress Scale
data collection/input, procedure for,
  54–56, 55*b*
Davies, Claire, 59*b*, 91*b*, 115*b*, 130*b*, 134*b*
deep-tissue wound injuries, 46
dependent variables, 77, 126, 127*b*
descriptive research designs, 77
  goal of, 82
  types of, 82–83
    case studies, 84, 84*b*
    correlational designs, 84–85
    explanatory research designs, 83–84, 84*b*
    exploratory research designs, 83, 83*b*
descriptive statistical analysis, 59, 59*b*, 123,
  142–146, 143–144*t*, 145*f*
diagnostic odds ratio (DOR), 113, 114*b*
disseminating findings
  assumptions, 149–151
  journal's perspective, 163, 164*f*
    editor responds to an inquiry, 165
    editor's decision to reject/forward for
      review, 165–166
    letter/email message to editor, 165, 165*b*
    peer reviewers, role of, 166

    requests for revisions, 166–167
    response to authors, 166
  research consultant's role, 151
    abstracts, 151–153, 152*t*, 153*b*
    internal reports, 151, 152*b*
    transforming practice into publication,
      research-friendly environment's
      guide, 153
    collaborative writing, 160–161, 162*b*
    developing manuscript, 157–158, 158*b*
    evaluating rigor of design, 156–157, 157*b*
    journal submission, 161
    preparing early for publication, 154–155,
      155–156*b*
    response to request for revisions,
      162–163, 162*t*
    selecting journal, 158–160, 160*b*
dissemination of findings, 30, 35, 61
  organizational policy publication,
    delineated, 62–69, 62–68*t*, 69*b*
Distress Anxiety Stress Scale (DASS), 102*b*
DOR. *See* diagnostic odds ratio
double-blinded randomized controlled trials,
  79, 80*b*

E

EBP. *See* evidence-based practice
EBP projects, 13–15
  Iowa Model of Evidence-Based Practice,
    13–14
  Johns Hopkins Nursing Evidence-Based
    Practice Model, 14–15
  strategies used to access, 11–12*t*
editors
  decision to reject/forward for review,
    165–166
  letter/email message to, 165, 165*b*
  response to inquiry, 165
  response to authors, 166
educational intervention, 53–54
educational offerings, 31
Edwards, John, 80*b*
email message to editor, 165, 165*b*
errors, 108–109
ethnography, 92
evidence-based practice (EBP)
  achieving, 7–9
  benefits and barriers, 2–3, 2*b*
  defined, 7
  gathering evidence, 9
  methods, 10–13. *See also specific methods*
    EBP projects, 13–15
    quality improvement, 15–17

research process, 17, 18*b*
    similarities and differences among, 11–12*t*
    support for, 2–3, 2*b*
exclusion criteria, 87
exercise, effect of music on, 158*b*
experimental research designs, 78–79
    advantages, 79–80
    disadvantages, 80–81
explanatory research designs, 83–84, 84*b*
exploration phase, Research-Friendly
        Environment Model
    caregiver's idea, 45–47, 47*b*
    initial research question, 48–50, 49*b*
    literature review, 47–48
exploratory research designs, 83, 83*b*
external validity, 77

F

face-to-face interviews, 52, 85–86, 117
face validity, 109
Fisher's least, 137
formulation phase, Research-Friendly
        Environment Model, 50–51
    data collection/input, procedure for,
        54–56, 55*b*
    intervention, 53–54
    measures, 51–53, 52*b*
    variables, 51, 52*b*
frequency distribution, 142–146
Fultz, Allison, 59*b*, 146*b*
funding for research, 39, 40–41*t*

G

G power, 131
generalizability, 77
generous leadership, 27, 30
    activities, 30–33, 32*b*
GPA. *See* Grade Point Average
Grade Point Average (GPA), 184
Groppo-Lawless, Sarah, 153*b*
grounded theory, 91–92

H

Hahn, Jeri, 52*b*, 102*b*, 155*b*
Hawthorne effect, 81
HBMM. *See* Hospital-Based Measurement
        Model

healthcare system, changes in, 4
homogeneity, 108
    of variance, 132
Honaker, Jeremy, 49*b*, 84*b*, 116*b*, 133*b*
Honaker Suspected Deep-Tissue Injury
        Severity Scale (HSDTISS), 18, 116
Hospital-Based Guide to Statistical Analysis,
        124, 125*f*
Hospital-Based Measurement Model
        (HBMM)
    measurement, 97–98, 97*f*
        administering instrument, 116–117
        developing instrument, 103–115
        literature review, 99–101
        modifing existing instrument, 101–102
        need for, 98–99
        select instrument from literature,
            101, 102*b*
hospital culture, 170–171
hourly rounding, 35*b*
HSDTISS. *See* Honaker Suspected Deep-
        Tissue Injury Severity Scale
"huddle" process, 103
hypothesis testing, 112

I

ICC. *See* intraclass correlation coefficient
inclusion criteria, 87
independence, assumption of, 133, 140
independent variables, 77, 126, 127*b*
inferential statistical analysis, 59–61, 123, 131
    nonparametric statistical tests, 139,
        140*b*, 141*t*
        difference, 140–142, 141*f*, 141*t*
    parametric statistics
        assumptions of, 132–133
        correlational statistical tests,
            133–134, 134*b*
        prediction, 137–139, 139*b*
        relationship, 133, 133*b*
        statistical tests for difference, 134–136,
            135–136*b*
        testing mean differences among more
            than two groups, 136–137, 137–138*b*
        testing mean differences between two
            groups, 134
institutional review board (IRB), 36, 171–172
    approval, 57
interaction, meaning of, 136
internal consistency, 115
internal reports, 151, 152*b*
internal validity, 82
Internet, 117

interrater reliability, 115, 116*b*
interval data, 127, 132
intraclass correlation coefficient (ICC), 134
Iowa Model of Evidence-Based Practice, 13–14
IRB. *See* institutional review board
items, 103
    closed-ended items, 105, 105–106*b*
    open-ended items, 104

J

Johns Hopkins Nursing Evidence-Based
    Practice Model, 14–15
journal
    citation reports, 159
    editors
        decision to reject/forward for review,
            165–166
        letter/email message to, 165, 165*b*
        responds to an inquiry, 165
    peer reviewers, role of, 166
    requests for revisions, 166–167
    response to authors, 166
    selecting, 158–160, 160*b*
    submission, 161

K

Kentucky Virtual Library (KYVL), 37
Kjelland, Kim, 47*b*, 105–106*b*, 140*b*
knee arthroplasty, 80*b*
Kruskal-Wallis test, 141–142
KYVL. *See* Kentucky Virtual Library

L

laboratory for caregiver-initiated research, 173
leadership
    Baptist Health Lexington Grid, 27, 28–29*t*
    generous leadership, 27, 30
        activities, 30–33, 32*b*
    influence of, 26–27
Lean Six Sigma process, 16
Lengerich, Alex, 100*b*, 110*b*
letter to editor, 165, 165*b*
levels of evidence, 9–10*t*
levels of measurement, 127–128, 128*b*
Lewis, Debra, 18*b*, 107*b*, 162*b*
Lewis, Preston, 69*b*, 88*b*, 129*b*
librarians, 37–38

Likert scale, 107–108
literature review, 47–48, 99–101
literature searching, 37–38

M

Magnet designation, 4–5
    increasing expectations, 169–170
Magnet Hospital Recognition Program for
    Excellence in Nursing Services, 4
main effect, meaning of, 136
manipulation of variable, 77
Mann-Whitney U test, 140
manuscript. *See also* journal
    developing, 157–158, 158*b*
    for publication, 62, 68
McCowan, Denise, 10*b*, 83*b*, 152*b*
means, 128–129
measurement, 85–87
    Hospital-Based Measurement Model, 97–98
        administering instrument, 116–117
        developing instrument, 103–115
        literature review, 99–101
        modifing existing instrument, 101–102
        need for, 98–99
        select instrument from literature, 101, 102*b*
        testing of instruments developed for use
            across settings, 119*t*, 120
measures
    comparison of, 112
    criteria for assessing
        construct, 111–112
        content, 109–111
        criterion-related, 112–113
    criteria for evaluating scientific usefulness
        of, 108–109
    identification of, 51–53, 52*b*
    self-report, 96
medians, 128–129
"mentoring" strategy, 31
modes, 128–129
Moe, Krista, 136*b*
multicollinearity, 138
multiple regression, 138

N

Neuroscience Nursing Research Center
    Fellowship Model, 176*t*, 177–178,
    180–182
nominal data, 106, 107*b*, 127
nonlibrarian as contact person, 37

nonparametric statistical tests, 123, 139
   difference, 140–142, 141f, 141t
norm-referenced measures, 96
normal distribution, 132
null hypothesis, 129
Nurse Research Internship, 185–186
Nurse Scholars Strategy, 184–185
Nursing Fellowship Program, 176t, 178,
   180–182
nursing practice, 5–6

O

odds ratio, 138–139
   diagnostic, 113, 114b
open-ended items, 104
ordinal data, 127
organizational policy publication, delineated,
   62–69, 62–68t

P

parametric statistics, 123
   assumptions of, 132–133
   correlational statistical tests, 133–134
   prediction, 137–139
   relationship, 133
   statistical tests for difference, 134–136
   testing mean differences among more than
      two groups, 136–137
   testing mean differences between two
      groups, 134
patient care, changing expectations, 170
Patient Protection and Affordable Care Act
   (ACA), 4
Peanut Ball, influence of, 8
Pearson Product Moment, 133
Pearson's chi-square test, 139
peer reviewers, role of, 166
PET model. See Practice question, Evidence,
   and Translation (PET) model
phenomenology, 91, 91b
point-biserial correlation coefficient, 134
post-mastectomy compression garment, 78b
power analysis, 130–131, 131b
Practice question, Evidence, and Translation
   (PET) model, 15
preliminary instrument, 108
profession of nursing, future directions, 175
professional development, 31
psychological well-being, 100, 100b
publication, preparing for, 154–155, 155–156b

Q

qualitative research, 8–9
   assumptions underlying, 89–90
   types of, 90–91
      ethnography, 92
      grounded theory, 91–92
      phenomenology, 91, 91b
quality improvement
   defined, 15
   Lean Six Sigma process, 16–17
   projects, 16
   strategies used to access, 11–12t
quantitative research, 8, 76–77
   assumptions underlying, 77
   designs, 77–78
      descriptive research designs, 82–85
      experimental research designs, 78–81, 78b
      quasi-experimental research designs,
         76, 81–82
   measurement, 85–87
   sample size, 87–88, 88b
   selection, 87–88
quasi-experimental research designs, 76
   advantages, 81
   disadvantages, 82
questioning, encouraging, 30, 170

R

randomized controlled trials (RCTs), 76–77,
   78–79, 156
   advantages, 79–80
   disadvantages, 80–81
rank data, 140, 141t
ratio, 127
ratio data, 132
RCTs. See randomized controlled trials
readmissions, reasons for, 152b
regression analysis, 137–138
relationship, 133, 133b
reliability, 98, 114
repeated measures ANOVA (RMANOVA),
   137, 138b
research
   attitudes toward, 171
   defined, 17
   funding for, 39, 40–41t
research consultants, 30, 33–35, 35b
   goal of, 160
   role in disseminating findings, 151
      abstracts, 151–153, 152t, 153b
      internal reports, 151, 152b

Research Consultation Model, 177*t*, 179–182
research designs, 77–78
    descriptive research designs, 82–85
    experimental research designs, 78–81, 78*b*
    quasi-experimental research designs, 81–82
research-friendly environment (RFE)
    in acute care setting. *See* acute care setting,
        research-friendly environment in
    strategies to assist in development of, 175,
        175–176*t*. *See also specific strategies*
        desired outcomes, similarities, 181
        expectations, differences, 181
        expertise involved, similarities, 182
        formality of offerings, differences, 181
        participant identification, differences,
            180–181
        rationale for strategies, similarities, 181
        teaching/learning methods,
            differences, 181
Research-Friendly Environment Model
        (RFEM), 6, 43, 44*f*
    analysis
        content analysis, 58
        descriptive statistical analysis, 59
        inferential statistical analysis, 59–61
    application, 56–57
        institutional review board approval, 57
    dissemination, 61
        organizational policy publication,
            delineated, 62–69, 62–68*t*
    exploration
        caregiver's idea, 45–47, 47*b*
        initial research question, 48–50, 49*b*
        literature review, 47–48
    formulation, 50–51
        data collection/input, procedure for,
            54–56
        intervention, 53–54
        measures, identification of, 51–53
        variables, identification of, 51
    research group/council, 30–31
    research hypothesis, 129
    research methods. *See* qualitative research;
        quantitative research
    research process, 17, 18*b*
        strategies used to access, 11–12*t*. *See also
        specific strategies*
    research question, initial, 48–50, 49*b*
    Research Training Program for Point-of-Care
        Clinicians, 176*t*, 179, 180–182
    resources
        recommendation for future, 171–172
        research-friendly environment
            funding for research, 39, 40–41*t*
            institutional review board, role of, 36
            librarians, role of, 37–38

research consultants, 33–35, 35*b*
    staffing resource, 38, 39*t*
reviewers
    response to authors, 166
    role of, 166
revisions
    requests for revisions, 166–167
    response to request for, 162–163, 162*t*
RFE. *See* research-friendly environment
RFEM. *See* Research-Friendly
        Environment Model
rigor of design, evaluating, 156–157, 157*b*
RM ANOVA. *See* repeated measures ANOVA

S

sample selection, 87
sample size, 87–88, 88*b*
scale development, 106–108
Schreiber, Judith, 55*b*, 135*b*, 157*b*
self-report measures, 96
sensitivity, calculations of, 113
Sheffe test, 137
significance level (p value), 140
significance, meaning of, 60
simple linear regression, 138
Six Sigma process, 16
Spearman's rho, 142
specificity, calculations of, 113
Speech-Language-Hearing Association, 153
SPSS. *See* Statistical Package for the Social
        Sciences
staffing resource, annual costs for, 38, 39*t*
statistical analysis, answering questions,
        123–124
    computer software, 124
    descriptive statistics, 142–146, 143–144*t*,
        145–146*b*, 145*f*
    inferential statistics. *See* inferential
        statistical analysis
    statistical terms and concepts,
        124–125, 125*f*
        confidence intervals, 130, 130*b*
        independent and dependent variables,
            126, 127*b*
        levels of measurement, 127–128, 128*b*
        means, medians, and modes, 128–129
        power analysis, 130–131, 131*b*
        statistical significance, 128, 129*b*
        type I and type II errors, 129
        variables, 125–126, 126*b*
Statistical Package for the Social Sciences
        (SPSS), 124
statistical significance, 128, 129*b*

Stefaniak, Karen, 175*b*
Stoltz, Regina, 32*b*, 81*b*, 128, 138*b*
success, acknowledging, 30

T

telephone interviews, 117
test–retest approach, 114
Thompson, Melanie, 2*b*, 19*b*, 126*b*
timing of publication, 159
transforming practice into publication
    research-friendly environment's guide, 153
        collaborative writing, 160–161, 162*b*
        developing manuscript, 157–158, 158*b*
        evaluating rigor of design, 156–157,
            157*b*
        journal submission, 161
        preparing early for publication, 154–155,
            155–156*b*
        response to request for revisions, 162–
            163, 162*t*
        selecting journal, 158–160, 160*b*
transitory personal factors, 109
tuition reimbursement program, 31
Tussey, Kathy, 160*b*
type I errors, 129
type II errors, 129

V

validity, 98. *See also* external validity; internal
        validity
    construct, 111–112
    content, 109–111
    criterion-related, 112–113

value systems, 89
variables, 125–126, 126*b*
    defined, 95
    identification of, 51, 52*b*
visual analogue scales (VAS), 107

W

Watson's Theory of Human Caring, 25–26
Weyl, Holly, 2*b*, 127*b*
Wheeler, Peggy, 78*b*
Wilcoxon rank sum test, 140
Wilcoxon signed rank test, 141
writing process, 160–161

Y

Yackzan, Susan, 102*b*

Z

z score, 140